UNDERSTANDING THE HEART
& ITS DISEASES

McGraw-Hill Series in Health Education

DEOBOLD B. VAN DALEN, Consulting Editor

COHEN   The Drug Dilemma
DALRYMPLE   Sex is for Real: Human Sexuality
    and Sexual Responsibility
DIEHL   Tobacco and Your Health: The Smoking
    Controversy
FORT   Alcohol: Our Biggest Drug Problem
MARTIN   Mental Health/Mental Illness:
    Revolution in Progress
ROSS and O'ROURKE   Understanding the Heart
    and its Diseases

UNDERSTANDING THE HEART & ITS DISEASES

John Ross, Jr., M.D.
School of Medicine
University of California, San Diego

Robert A. O'Rourke, M.D.
School of Medicine
University of California, San Diego

McGraw-Hill Book Company

New York St. Louis San Francisco Auckland Düsseldorf
Johannesburg Kuala Lumpur London Mexico Montreal
New Delhi Panama Paris São Paulo Singapore
Sydney Tokyo Toronto

To my wife, Lola Romanucci-Ross

UNDERSTANDING THE HEART AND ITS DISEASES

1 2 3 4 5 6 7 8 9 0 M U M U 7 9 8 7 6 5

Library of Congress Cataloging in Publication Data

Ross, John, date
   Understanding the heart and its diseases.

   (McGraw-Hill series in health education)
   Includes index.
   1. Heart—Diseases. 2. Heart. I. O'Rourke,
Robert A., joint author. II. Title.
[DNLM: 1. Heart diseases. WG200 R824u]
RC672.R643   616.1'2   75-11529
ISBN 0-07-053861-1
ISBN 0-07-053862-X pbk.

This book was set in Times Roman by Black Dot, Inc.
The editors were Richard R. Wright and David Dunham;
the production supervisor was Judi Allen.
The cover drawing was done by Stephen Sprung.
The Murray Printing Company was printer and binder.

Contents

Preface   ix

1 Circulation of the Blood   1
The Two Circulations of the Body   3
Arterial Blood Pressure and the Circulation to the
  Body   3
The Capillaries   7
The Veins of the Body   8
The Lung (pulmonary) Circulation   8
The Pathway of a Red Blood Cell   9

**2 The Subsystems of the Heart and Regulation of the
   Circulation**   12
The Heart's Subsystems   13
  The valves of the heart   13
  The electrical pacemaker and conduction system   15
  The coronary arteries   17
  The heart muscle   17

The Nervous Regulation of the Heartbeat and
   Circulation   20
Starling's Law of the Heart   23

3 **Diagnosing Heart Disease**   25
The Physical Examination   26
The Electrocardiogram   29
   What type of information is contained in the
      electrocardiogram?   30
   The exercise electrocardiogram   33
The Phonocardiogram   33
The Echocardiogram   34
Cardiac Catheterization and Angiocardiography   35
   What can be accomplished through the cardiac
      catheter?   39

4 **Role of General Factors in Cause, Prevention, and
   Treatment of Heart Disease**   44
Obesity   45
Diets   46
Exercise   50
Smoking   52
Sexual Activity   53
Alcohol and the Heart   54
The Heart of the Athlete   55
Emotional Stress   56
Pregnancy   57
Drug Abuse   59

5 **Diseases of the Heart Valves**   62
Rheumatic Fever   63
Effects of Valvular Damage   64
Narrowing of the Mitral Valve (Mitral Stenosis)   65
Leakage of the Mitral Valve (Mitral Insufficiency or
   Regurgitation)   67
Narrowing of the Aortic Valve (Aortic Stenosis)   67
Leakage of the Aortic Valve (Aortic Regurgitation
   or Insufficiency)   69
Right-Sided Valve Disease   69
The Medical Treatment of Valvular Heart Disease   69
Blood Clots   70

6   Diseases of the Electrical System: Heart Rhythm
       Disorders and Heart Block   73
     Extra Beats   76
     Rapid Heart Rhythms   78
     Electric Countershock   82
     Slow Heart Rhythms   83
     Electronic Pacemakers   85

7   Diseases of the Coronary Arteries: Chest Pain and
       Heart Attack   88
     The Cause of Coronary Artery Disease   89
     Risk Factors   90
     The Symptoms and Mechanism of Heart Pain
       (Angina Pectoris)   92
     The Symptoms and Mechanism of a Heart Attack
       ("Myocardial Infarction")   95
     The Treatment of Coronary Heart Disease   97
        Management of the "coronary prone" individual   98
        Patterns and treatment of elevated cholesterol and
           triglycerides in the blood   99
        The medical treatment of chest pain   103
        The treatment of heart attack   105

8   High Blood Pressure   109
     The Normal Blood Pressure   109
     Causes of High Blood Pressure   111
     Hormones and High Blood Pressure   113
     How is High Blood Pressure Detected?   115
     Complications of High Blood Pressure   115
     Treatment of High Blood Pressure   117
     Does Lowering Blood Pressure Reduce Risk?   119

9   Heart Failure and Diseases of Heart Muscle   121
     The Causes of Heart Failure   121
     The Treatment of Heart Failure   127
     Prevention of Heart Failure   129

10 Inborn Heart Disease   132
     Narrowing or Constriction of a Blood Vessel or
       Heart Valve   134
     Abnormal Holes or Communications in the Heart   138

Ventricular Septal Defect and Pulmonic Valve
  Narrowing (Tetralogy of Fallot)   140
Abnormal Connections of the Large Blood Vessels
  Leading to or from the Heart   141

11 **Heart Surgery**   144
    Early Attempts at Heart Surgery   144
    Heart-Lung Machines   146
    Valve Replacement   147
    Surgery for Congenital Heart Disease   150
    Surgery of Coronary Artery Disease   151
    Heart Transplantation   154
    Assisted Circulation and the Artificial Heart   156

Glossary   159

Index   173

Preface

This book has been written primarily to provide the student of the health sciences and the lay person with sufficiently detailed information about the structure and function of the heart and circulation to allow a working understanding of heart disease. The four main subsystems of the heart—its valves, electrical system, muscular walls, and coronary arteries—are used as the basis for describing the effects of common diseases such as high blood pressure and coronary occlusion (heart attack). The reader will learn how physicians can diagnose heart disease by listening to the heart, as well as by special techniques such as the exercise electrocardiogram, heart (cardiac) catheterization, and coronary arteriography. Although not intended primarily as a manual for heart patients, the book also indicates the rationale behind the use of various heart medications, and the role of heart surgery in treating major heart problems—valvular, coronary, and inborn, or congenital, heart disease. Finally, attention has been directed toward clarifying the role of various risk factors, such as obesity and smoking, and the importance of diet, exercise, alcohol, and other factors in modifying the course of heart disease. It may be hoped that with greater understanding of heart disease by the public, by students in the health sciences, by paramedical health professionals, and by heart patients and their families, we will be better able to improve measures for the prevention, early detection, and treatment of this leading cause of death in Western societies.

Acknowledgment

The excellent secretarial assistance of Ms. Hazel Wills is gratefully recognized.

Chapter 1

Circulation of the Blood

The first recorded observations on the heart and its function date back to Greece in the fifth and fourth centuries B.C., when the heart's chambers and its valves were described, along with the pulse rate and heart rhythm. But it was Galen, famous physician of Roman times (A.D. second century), who demonstrated not only the relation between the heartbeat and the pulse but also documented the fact that arteries contained blood and not air, as the Alexandrian school had taught for 400 years. Galen also described the heart and its three layers of fibers that he hesitated to call muscle. We know now, however, that the heart is indeed a remarkable, specialized muscle that functions with the help of a series of valves and its own electrical pacing system. After Galen, centuries passed before further major progress was forthcoming, although Leonardo daVinci and others made accurate drawings of the heart's anatomy.

William Harvey (1578–1657), an Englishman who had studied medicine at Padua, understood heart valve function and likened the heart's action to "2 clacks of a water bellows," an ancient wooden device which lifted water by means of primitive one-way valves. Harvey's great achievement was announced in 1628—the discovery of the circulation of the blood. The heart operates as one important link in a closed system of tubes, the blood vessels (composed of the arteries, capillaries, and veins), through which the blood cycles and recycles, and the elucidation of this simple fact was perhaps the most remarkable of all single discoveries concerning the circulation. Harvey deduced that capillaries, tiny blood vessels invisible to the naked eye, must exist and connect arteries to veins within the tissues. His deduction, remarkable because it took place before the discovery of the microscope made these minute vessels visible, was reached by observing the one-way flow of blood through the valves of the heart and circulation and measuring the actual volume of blood ejected by the heart in animal experiments. The direction of blood flow toward the tissues in the arteries and away from the tissues in the veins, made necessary by the one-way valves in the veins, together with the very large volume of flow (several gallons per minute—more than the whole circulation could possibly contain), led him to the correct conclusion: The blood must circulate around and around.

In the nineteenth century there was an efflorescence in the growth of information on the pathology of all forms of circulatory diseases, and the turn of the century saw the beginnings of the technology that has greatly increased the precision of our diagnosis of heart disease.

The physician specializing in heart disease (cardiologist) and the cardiovascular physiologist are interested in the minute details of structure and function of the heart's several components. It should be understood, however, that the sole function of this complex structure is to pump blood into the two major blood vessels which leave the heart, so that adequate blood flow, first to the lungs and then to the vital body organs, is maintained when we are at rest and made available in increased amounts during various forms of stress. This blood carries nutriments (amino acids, fats, sugar), oxygen (a fuel important to the life processes of all cells in the body), and waste products from the tissues to the lungs and kidneys for elimination. The heart has an extraordinary ability to contract continuously over many years and to accept and pump out whatever quantity of blood returns to it; during strenuous muscular exercise, for example, the demands for fuel of the muscles of the limbs may call on the heart to rapidly increase its output of blood as much as tenfold. Not only must the heart pump blood to other vital organs in the body, but it also must supply blood to *itself* through its own nourishing blood vessels, the coronary arteries. We shall first consider how the heart and its components function under normal circumstances, since various forms of human disease are associated with disorders in their structure and function.

The Two Circulations of the Body

Basically, the heart consists of two pumps which supply two separate circulations, that to the lungs and that supplying the remainder of the body. As shown in Figure 1-1, the left-sided pumping chamber (left ventricle) is a thick-walled muscular chamber responsible for pumping blood to the main circulation, that is, first to the arteries and then to the veins that reach most of the body. The right-sided pumping chamber (right ventricle) pumps blood to a second circulation having a completely separate set of arteries and veins serving only the lungs (Figure 1-1, stippled areas). In addition, the heart has two small receiving chambers which act as "booster pumps" and are termed the "atria." The left atrium, which receives oxygenated red blood from the lungs, is a thin-walled muscular chamber situated just behind the main left pumping chamber, and it contracts just prior to the left ventricle, thereby helping to fill it. The right atrium, similarly situated behind the right ventricle (Figure 1-1), receives blue, venous blood from the large veins which drain the body.

Arterial Blood Pressure and the Circulation to the Body

The oxygenated red blood that flows through the arteries to most of the body leaves the heart by way of a single large vessel, the aorta. This vessel arises directly from the left ventricle and then

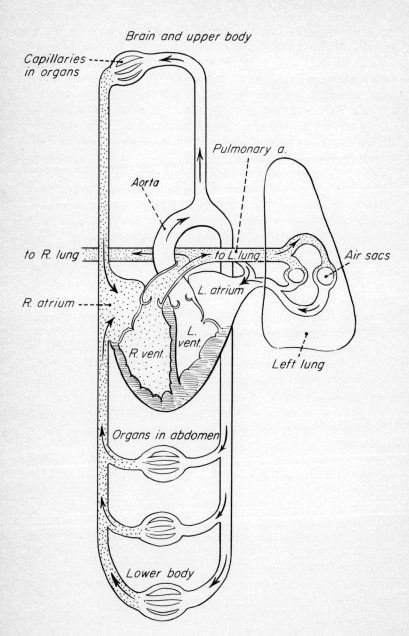

Brain and upper body

Capillaries in organs

Pulmonary a.

Aorta

to R. lung   to L. lung   Air sacs

R. atrium

L. atrium

L. vent.

R. vent.

Left lung

Organs in abdomen

Lower body

branches to supply all the organs of the body (Figure 1-1). When an individual is in an upright position, as we are during most of the day, there is a column of blood contained in the arteries which supply the upper portion of the body and the head that extends about 25 inches in height above the heart (Figure 1-1). Therefore, the left-sided pump (left ventricle) must generate sufficient pressure to lift this blood column with each heartbeat. It also must develop sufficient extra pressure within the main arteries to force blood forward through all the various organs of the body. Therefore, this left-sided pumping chamber has a thick muscular wall which allows it to generate a high pressure in the systemic arteries. By laying a finger on the pulse at the inner side of your wrist near the base of the thumb, or in your neck at the angle of the jaw, it is possible to feel the pulse of blood as it moves through the arteries each time the left ventricle contracts. You may notice that it requires considerable pressure with your fingertip over the artery at your wrist to abolish the pulse. Indeed, in the normal person the pressure in a pneumatic cuff must be inflated to above 130 millimeters of mercury (or 3 pounds per square inch) to abolish the pulse. As the pressure in such an inflated cuff is then slowly reduced, it is the sound of the blood as it first begins to pass under the cuff with each heartbeat that the physician hears through the stethoscope while listening over the artery in the arm (Figure 1-2). At that moment the pressure in the cuff is observed on a dial. This pressure is the *systolic* blood pressure (the highest pressure during each pulse). As the pressure in the cuff is lowered further, a muffling of the sound occurs as the blood begins to rush continuously beneath the cuff, and at this point the dial is read again to give another (lower) pressure, the *diastolic* blood pressure. Thus, the blood pressure is generally

Figure 1-1 Overall scheme of the heart and circulation. The two separate pumping chambers of the heart, the right ventricle (R. vent.) and the left ventricle (L. vent.), serve to pump blood into the lungs and the body through two large blood vessels: The vessel supplying the lungs is the pulmonary artery (Pulmonary a.), and that supplying the body is the aorta. There are two receiving chambers of the heart. The one receiving oxygenated blood from the lungs is the left atrium (L. atrium), and that receiving blood from the veins of the body (blue blood in the veins is stippled) is the right atrium (R. atrium). Branches from the aorta supply all the organs of the body. The blood flows in sequence through the right heart, the lungs, the left heart, and then to the body.

STEPS IN MEASUREMENT OF
BLOOD PRESSURE

1. CUFF INFLATED TO OCCLUDE ARTERY

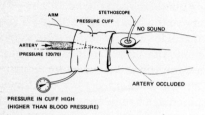

2. PRESSURE IN CUFF SLOWLY LOWERED

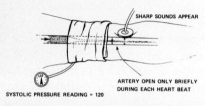

3. PRESSURE IN CUFF LOWERED FURTHER

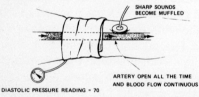

Figure 1-2 Method by which the blood pressure is taken using a standard pneumatic cuff on the arm (see text). Steps 1, 2, and 3 require initial inflation of the cuff so that the dial (lower left) reads a high pressure (well over 200 millimeters of mercury) and completely occludes the artery of the arm. The physician then listens with the stethoscope placed on the arm over the artery as the pressure in the cuff is slowly lowered (step 1); systolic pressure is then taken (step 2, in the example, 120 millimeters of mercury); and as the pressure is lowered further, the diastolic pressure is taken (step 3, in the example, 70 millimeters of mercury). The reading is then reported as 120 over 70.

expressed as two numbers, for example, 120 over 80 or 130/80 (a normal blood pressure). The level of diastolic pressure is determined primarily by how much resistance to flow (or degree of narrowing) exists in the small arteries of the various organs in the body. The diastolic pressure level has particular significance relative to high blood pressure (*hypertension*), because this disease usually involves initially the blood vessels rather than the heart; that is, an abnormally *high resistance* to blood flow is present in the small arteries of the systemic circulation. Therefore, the diastolic pressure is elevated during the relaxation phase of the heart cycle, and the heart must also generate an increased systolic pressure to drive the blood forward through the abnormally narrowed vessels. Prolonged high blood pressure can, of course, have detrimental secondary effects on the heart, kidneys, brain, and other organs. (See Chapter 8.)

The Capillaries

Within the various organs, the small arteries ultimately divide into many tiny thin-walled blood vessels, the capillaries, from which oxygen and various nutriments are exchanged and waste products taken up. Capillaries are also found within the lungs. The capillaries are the smallest blood vessels in the body and also the most numerous. They measure about 0.5 millimeter in length and are hardly more than the size of one red blood cell in diameter. The number of capillaries in some organs is enormous; in the heart, for example, there are as many as 5,000 capillaries per square millimeter of heart muscle. Because of their large number, the surface area of these thin-walled vessels is very great, and the velocity of blood flow through them is low. Compared to the large artery, the aorta, through which all the blood leaving the heart must pass, the cross-sectional area of the capillaries is 800 times greater; this means that the rate of blood flow through these tiny vessels is about 800 times slower than in the aorta. All these factors, the tremendous surface area, the slow rate of blood flow, and the thin walls of these vessels, make the capillaries a highly favorable site for the exchange of gases (oxygen and carbon dioxide) and nutriments (such as amino acids and carbohydrates) within the tissues. Large protein molecules contained in the bloodstream, however, cannot pass through the walls of the capillaries. As the oxygen is removed for use by the organs, the pigment hemoglobin within the red blood cells changes color, and consequently the blood turns a darker red, or "blue." This "venous" blood then enters small veins, which converge to form larger and larger vessels, finally entering two major veins which return the venous blood to the right-sided receiving chamber of the heart (Figure 1-1).

The Veins of the Body

The veins drain the body and its internal organs. These thin-walled vessels normally carry blood at a low pressure (5 or 6 millimeters of mercury, compared to the 130 millimeters of mercury in the major arteries). While blood flowing in the arteries of the arm, for example, is flowing *away* from the heart, after it passes through the tiny capillaries it passes into the veins and flows *toward* the heart. Contained within the veins of the arms and legs are a series of one-way valves.

It is a simple matter to demonstrate the action of a one-way valve such as those within the heart or in a vein. Keep in mind that venous blood returns through the veins from the fingertips and flows up the arm toward the heart. Hold one of your arms in a lowered position and then apply the index finger of your other hand to one of the veins on the back of your hand near the wrist. By applying gentle pressure to the vein and moving your finger away from your wrist toward your fingers, you will notice that at some point along the course of the vein there is a valve which prevents blood from flowing backward towards the fingers; as you continue to move your finger along the vein, it remains empty. When the finger is lifted, blood can be seen to flow forward and the valve opens. It is when these valves in the veins become leaky and insufficient that varicose veins of the legs are observed.

The Lung (Pulmonary) Circulation

The second circulation of the body is not accessible to direct examination because it lies entirely within the chest cavity. This circulation carries blood only to and from the lungs (in Latin, *pulmos*) and is termed the "pulmonary" circulation. A single major blood vessel (the pulmonary artery) carries the venous blood from the right ventricle (Figure 1-1), branches into smaller and smaller pulmonary arteries, finally ending in delicate capillaries which surround the millions of tiny air sacs within the lungs. Through the thin walls of these lung capillaries, oxygen is taken up and carbon dioxide released. The bright red, oxygenated blood then passes into veins (the pulmonary veins) which connect to the left-sided receiving chamber (the left atrium). The left ventricle is then filled and pumps the oxygenated blood around again to the major arteries of the body, completing the circuit.

The right heart and pulmonary circulation differ in several ways from the left heart and systemic circulation. The lung arteries and capillaries offer little resistance to blood flow, and since the lungs are at about the same height in the body as the heart, the right ventricle need not develop nearly as high a pressure as the left ventricle (indeed, the average pressure is only one-sixth that in the left ventricle, or approximately 20 millimeters of mercury). As a consequence, although the right ventricle must pump the same volume of blood per minute as the left ventricle (the two pumps operate within a closed circuit) it does not work as hard, and its muscular wall normally is only one-fourth as thick as that of the left ventricle (Figure 1-1).

The Pathway of a Red Blood Cell

If we were to trace the course of a red blood cell as it moves with the bloodstream within a vein, it first passes into the chest and toward the heart through one of the large veins draining the upper and lower parts of the body. Next, it passes through the small receiving chamber (atrium) on the right side and then enters the right-sided pumping chamber (right ventricle). During contraction of the heart, the right ventricle pumps the red cell into the blood vessels which supply the lungs, from whence it courses through increasingly smaller branching vessels which finally reach the tiny, thin-walled vessels (capillaries) surrounding the air sacs in the lung. There, oxygen contained in the air diffuses through the wall of the air sac and the wall of the capillary to enter the blood plasma and then the red blood cell, to combine with hemoglobin. The protein pigment hemoglobin binds oxygen and allows each red blood cell to store and transport large amounts of oxygen. Also, within these capillaries carbon dioxide (a waste product from tissue metabolism) diffuses out of the red cell and into the air sacs to be exhaled. Within the moving bloodstream the red blood cell then passes into the progressively larger veins which drain the lungs into the left-sided receiving chamber of the heart and from there enters the left-sided

pumping chamber (left ventricle). Again, during contraction of
the heart, the blood is expelled by the left ventricle into the major
artery leading from the heart (the aorta) from whence it enters
progressively smaller arteries supplying the organs of the body.
Ultimately it reaches *another* set of capillaries, which lie within
tissues of the various organs. Here, as in the lung, because of the
tremendous increase in cross-sectional area within the capillary
portion of the vascular bed, the blood flow becomes quite slow.
Oxygen from the red blood cell is given up (as are other
nutriments contained in the blood) and diffuses to the tissues
where it is used for tissue metabolism. The red blood cell changes
to a dark color (responsible for the bluish hue of blood in the
veins of the body) and takes up carbon dioxide. The blood then
drains into the veins leading from the organ into larger veins and
ultimately courses back to the right side of the heart and back
again to the lungs for reoxygenation, thereby completing the
cycle.

Knowledge of the nature of the two circulations of the body
permits an understanding of the effects of blood clots which may
form in the circulation. Clots that are formed in the veins of the
body, usually in diseased veins in the legs, travel through the right
side of the heart and lodge in branches of the pulmonary artery.
Such clots cannot reach the rest of the body because they cannot
pass through the tiny capillaries of the lung (Figure 1-1).* On the
other hand, clots that form in the left-sided chambers of the heart
or the arteries of the body, when dislodged, travel directly to the
vital organs of the body (brain, kidneys, etc.) and may cause
blockage of blood flow with serious damage.

REFERENCES

General

Blakeslee, A., and Stamler, J., *Your Heart Has Nine Lives*, Prentice-
Hall, Inc., Englewood Cliffs, N.J., 1966.

*A very large blood clot which reaches the lung (a pulmonary embolus) may cause
severe distress by blocking blood flow through the lung and may constitute a medical
emergency. Such clots usually originate when inflammation and clot formation
(thrombophlebitis) occur in the veins of the leg.

The Heart and Blood Vessels (E. M. 603), American Heart Association, New York, 1973 (pamphlet).*

Willius, F. A., and Keys, T. E., *Cardiac Classics*, Mosby, St. Louis, 1941.

Scientific Works

Braunwald, E., Ross, J. Jr., and Sonnenblick, E. H.: "Mechanisms of Contraction of the Normal and Failing Heart," *New England Journal of Medicine* **227**:794–800, 853–863, 910–920, 962–971, 1012–1022, 1967.

Braunwald, E., Ross, J. Jr., and Sonnenblick, E. H.: *Mechanisms of Contraction of the Normal and Failing Heart*, 2d ed., Little, Brown and Company, Boston, 1975.

Netter, F. H.: *The Ciba Collection of Medical Illustrations, Volume 5, Heart*, Ciba Pharmaceutical Company, Summit, N.J., 1969.

*This pamphlet and other American Heart Association pamphlets can be obtained from your local Heart Association or by writing the American Heart Association, 44 East 23rd Street, New York, New York 10010.

The Subsystems of the Heart and Regulation of the Circulation

The heart's contraction depends on the perfectly synchronized operation of four major "subsystems." Each of these is subject to certain diseases that can profoundly affect the heart's function. These four functional components consist of

1 The valves of the heart
2 The electrical pacemaker and conduction system
3 The coronary arteries
4 The heart muscle

We will first consider the normal structure and function of these components and then will elaborate on their role in specific diseases of the heart in later chapters.

THE HEART'S SUBSYSTEMS

The Valves of the Heart

The pumping chamber, or ventricle, contracts or squeezes (like the opening and closing of a fist) to eject the blood contained within it. If there were no valves in the heart, the blood could go in two directions, forward into the artery and backward into the atrium, but the valves at the entrance and exit to each ventricle allow the blood to flow forward. In addition, a series of valves, which prevent blood from flowing backward into the legs and arms when we are standing, is present within many of the systemic veins of the body. (See Chapter 1.)

The action of the valves within the heart permits blood to flow forward in only one direction. There are four heart valves, two on the right side and two on the left. Two of these valves lie directly below the large arteries that come from the right and left ventricles, and therefore they are called the "pulmonic" and "aortic" valves, respectively; these two valves prevent blood from running backward into the ventricles during their relaxation or filling phase, and they open during contraction of the ventricles to allow ejection of blood into the pulmonary artery and the aorta (Figure 2-1). The aortic valve serves a particularly important function, since when it is closed between each heart contraction, it allows a high pressure to be maintained in the aorta and its branch arteries. Thus blood flow to the vital organs can continue even while the ventricles are filling. The pulmonic valve serves a similar function relative to blood flow through the lungs (Figure 2-1).

While the above two valves are open, the remaining two heart valves are closed during the squeezing (contraction) phase of the heart cycle. Therefore, they prevent blood from leaking backward out of the ventricles as they eject blood forward, and they open, allowing blood to fill the ventricles during their relaxed phase between heartbeats. The tricuspid valve guards the entrance to the right ventricle (tricuspid, because it has three flexible leaflets), and the mitral valve (two leaflets) guards the left ventricle. As summarized diagrammatically in Figure 2-1, when

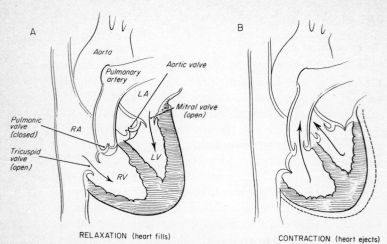

Figure 2-1 Cutaway view of the heart and the two large arteries leaving it which supply the lungs (pulmonary artery) and the remainder of the body (aorta). Two phases of the heart cycle are shown. In Panel *A* the phase of the heartbeat in which the heart is relaxed and filling is illustrated, and in Panel *B* the phase of the heart cycle in which the muscular walls of the heart contract causing blood to be ejected into the aorta and pulmonary artery is shown. In Panel *A* the two valves (mitral and tricuspid) that guard the entrances to the pumping chambers (the left ventricle, LV, and right ventricle, RV) are open to allow these chambers to fill from the receiving chambers (right atrium, RA, and left atrium, LA) when the heart is relaxed and filling. At the same time, the two valves guarding the entrance to the aortic and pulmonary valves are closed to prevent backward flow of blood from these two vessels into the heart. In Panel *B*, when the muscular wall of the pumping chamber shortens and ejects blood forward, the mitral and tricuspid valves snap shut to prevent backward flow of blood into the receiving chambers, while both the aortic and pulmonic valves are open to allow the forward flow of blood into the aorta and pulmonary artery.

the left ventricle contracts, the mitral valve closes and the aortic valve opens to allow ejection of blood; when the left ventricle relaxes, the aortic valve shuts to prevent backflow, and the mitral valve opens to allow filling of the ventricle from the left atrium. A similar sequence operates within the right ventricle.

The function of any one of these four valves can be severely affected by inborn heart defects, by bacterial infection of the valve, or by rheumatic heart disease that causes scarring of the valves. Obviously, if the valves leak or become narrowed, serious consequences can ensue for the heart and circulation (Chapter 5).

The Electrical Pacemaker and Conduction System

As shown in Figure 2-2, there is a small area of specialized tissue located in the wall of the right atrium called the "sinus node." Throughout life this tiny region continuously emits a series of electrical impulses at a rate of about seventy per minute when we are at rest. If a tiny electrode is placed inside a single heart muscle cell in this node, a small electrical potential can be measured across the membrane which surrounds the cell. The reason that the pacemaker cells in the sinus node automatically emit a series of electrical impulses is related to the fact that in these particular cells a continuous change occurs in the "leakiness" (permeability) of cell membrane during the resting phase after each impulse. Thus, the resting electrical potential slowly falls to a certain threshold level, at which point the cell automatically "fires" another electrical impulse. The electrical potential is then returned to its starting, resting stage by a process in which the cells use oxygen to pump ions (largely sodium) out of the cell's interior, and the cycle starts all over again.

Each electrical impulse spreads through the muscle of the right atrium and is then picked up by a special conducting system having a low electrical resistance that might be compared to a system of copper wires. This conducting system (Figure 2-2) begins at another "node," which lies at the junction between the two atria and the two ventricles (labeled "AV node" in Figure 2-2) and which briefly delays each electrical impulse and then sends it down the conducting fibers, which rapidly direct it to the muscle of the right and left ventricles. This electrical discharge causes the muscles of the heart to contract. The arrangement described is ideal for causing the atria to beat before the ventricles; it also assures that the two ventricles will contract together and respond together as the heart rate changes. Only the heart's pacemaker initiates the electrical signals. When the impulse arrives at each muscle cell of the heart, a resting electrical potential is reversed (depolarization) and the muscle cells are activated to contract.

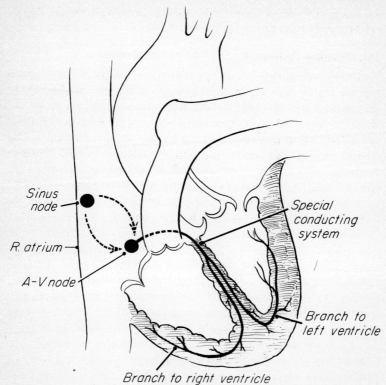

Figure 2-2 Diagram of the electrical conducting system of the heart. The pacemaker of the heart is situated in the right-sided receiving chamber, the right (R) atrium, and is called the "sinus node." Each heart cycle is started by an electrical impulse from the sinus node which travels over the receiving chambers and reaches another specialized group of cells called the AV node. This node delays the impulse and then sends it forward over specialized muscle fibers which serve as "wires." This special conducting system supplies branches to the two pumping chambers in order to provide electrical activation of the heart muscle for each heartbeat.

The electrical potentials from the heart can be recorded on the body's surface, and when the signal is amplified and inscribed on moving paper, the electrical events are readily visible as the electrocardiogram (Chapter 3). It is evident that disorders of the heart's pacemaker, or interruption of the special conducting pathways by disease processes, can seriously impair the ability of the heart to beat effectively (Chapter 6).

The Coronary Arteries

The heart is nourished with blood by the coronary arteries, which arise from the aorta (its first branches) just beyond the leaflets of the aortic valve (Figure 2-3). The left coronary artery divides into two branches, one going to the front and one to the side of the left ventricle, while the right coronary artery supplies blood to the right ventricle and also to the back of the left ventricle in most individuals. The coronary arteries break up into smaller and smaller branches which penetrate the wall of the heart and finally into tiny capillaries through which oxygen and nutriments are supplied to the heart muscle and to its electrical conduction system.

The heart is unique in that it is responsible for maintaining its own nourishment: It must maintain a sufficiently high pressure in the aorta to assure that an adequate amount of oxygenated blood is forced through the coronary arteries. If there is atherosclerotic (or arteriosclerotic) disease that causes narrowing of the coronary arteries, portions of the heart may not receive an adequate supply of blood even when the blood pressure is normal. An insufficient blood flow through these vital coronary arteries can cause chest pain, abnormal heart function, or even death of the heart muscle (heart attack) (Chapter 7) as well as disturbances of the heart's electrical activity.

The Heart Muscle

The means by which the muscle of the heart contracts is an interesting process, and over the past ten years an important story has emerged. In part it was made possible by the development of the electron microscope with its ability to magnify the structure of a single muscle cell tens of thousands of times. Basically, muscles are able to contract because two protein strands within the muscle interact chemically, a process which causes the strands or filaments to slide over one another. The two proteins, called actin and myosin, are grouped into small contracting units made up of many filaments, and many thousands of

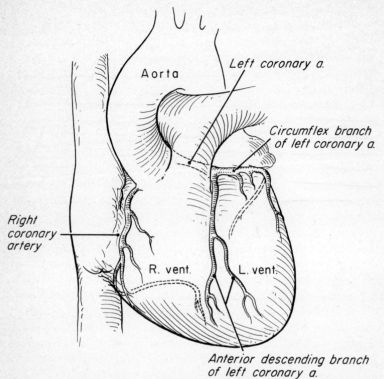

Figure 2-3 Outside view of the heart showing the blood vessels which supply the heart muscle: the coronary arteries (coronary a.). The two coronary arteries are the first branches from the aorta, arising just above the aortic valve. The right coronary artery passes over the surface of the heart giving branches to the right-sided pumping chamber, the right ventricle (R. vent.), and it usually passes around the heart to give a branch to the under surface of the left-sided pumping chamber, the left ventricle (L. vent.). The left coronary artery first passes behind the pulmonary artery and then divides into two branches, one of which supplies the front surface of the left ventricle (the anterior descending branch). The other branch encircles the heart to supply the side and back of the left ventricle (the circumflex branch). These coronary arteries send branches into the wall of the heart to supply oxygen and nutriments to the heart muscle.

these units are present in each muscle cell (Figure 2-4). As the electrical impulse travels over the muscle surface, it causes the ion calcium to be released from special sacs lying near the protein strands. The calcium is responsible for activating the contraction

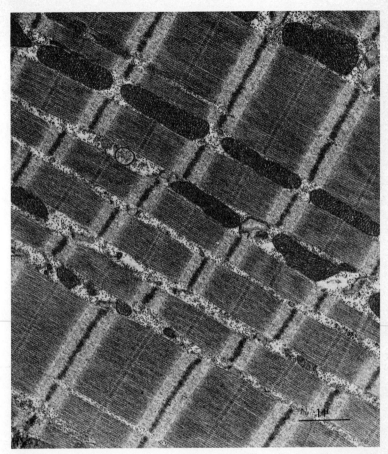

Figure 2-4   Electron micrograph of heart muscle at a magnification of about 10,000 times. The vertically arranged wide (dark) and narrow (light) band patterns represent arrays of many thick and thin protein strands, which slide in and out during each heartbeat (see Figure 2-5). The dark oval objects are mitochondria, which produce the energy (ATP) for muscle contraction.

process, and a series of chemical bonds is formed between the two sets of protein strands, the bonds strongly pulling one set of strands over the other much as two hairbrushes might be pushed together (see Figure 2-5). This process allows the muscles of the legs to lift weight or to work and the muscles of the heart to develop pressure and to propel blood. In the heart, the activating

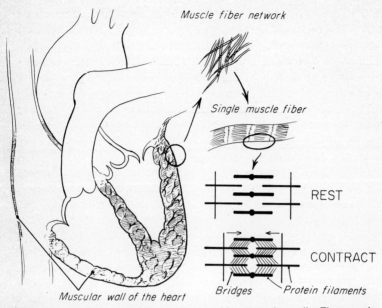

Figure 2-5 Diagram showing the heart and its muscular walls. The muscle of the pumping chambers is thick, particularly that of the left-sided pumping chamber; the relatively thin muscular wall of the receiving chambers also is shown. The circled insert from the wall of the left pumping chamber shows the muscle fiber network; each fiber is then magnified further to show its banded structure, as would be observed under the electron microscope (see Figure 2-4). The lower two diagrams on the right show how muscle contraction occurs: during the *rest* phase of the heart's cycle, the protein filaments in the muscle do not interact chemically but slide freely over one another. However, when the heart muscle is electrically activated to *contract*, the muscle fiber develops tension and shortens because chemical bridges are formed between the sets of protein filaments (actin and myosin), drawing the thin filaments inward much as if two hairbrushes were pushed together.

calcium returns to its storage site after each beat, and the heart relaxes until the next electrical impulse arrives.

THE NERVOUS REGULATION OF THE HEARTBEAT AND CIRCULATION

There are several hormonal substances which occur naturally in the body and are extremely important in helping to regulate the rate of the heart, the strength of the normal heartbeat, and the degree of contraction, or "resistance," in the small arteries of the body. Everyone recognizes that during emotional excitement (such as anger) or physical exercise, the heart rate becomes rapid, sometimes increasing from the normal value of 60 to 80 beats per minute to well over 200 beats per minute during strenuous exertion. In addition, one can often sense that the heart is "pounding," or beating more forcefully, and the blood pressure rises. Alternatively, during sleep, the heart may beat quietly at a rate as slow as fifty beats per minute. These normal variations in heart rate are summarized in Figure 2-6.

The three hormones that are responsible for these changes are epinephrine (sometimes called adrenalin), a related chemical substance called norepinephrine, and the compound acetylcholine. Epinephrine is released into the bloodstream directly from the adrenal glands (which lie in the abdomen near the kidneys) during emotional and physical stresses. Impulses from the central nervous system cause this release. This hormone, epinephrine, circulates within the bloodstream to reach the heart and arteries. Its action causes acceleration of the sinus node (increase in heart rate), more forceful contraction of the heart muscle, and contrac-

Figure 2-6 Diagrammatic representation of the variations in heart rate that may occur throughout the day during various activities in a normal individual.

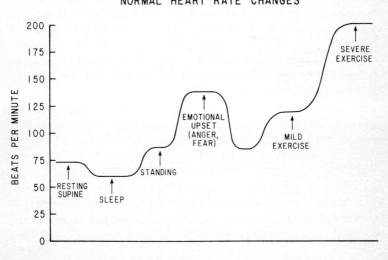

NORMAL HEART RATE CHANGES

tion of the muscle in the walls of some small arteries of the body; the latter provides an increased resistance to blood flow through these small blood vessels, and hence blood pressure is increased. In addition, throughout the heart muscle, and surrounding the heart's pacemaker and conduction system, is a network of special nerve fibers which contain the epinephrine-like compound norepinephrine. Similar nerve fibers containing norepinephrine also surround the small arteries of the body. When released from these nerve endings by nerve impulses from the central nervous system, norepinephrine (like epinephrine) increases the rate of the heart's pacemaker, causes the heart muscle to contract more forcefully, and constricts the small arteries.

A second, completely separate set of nerves also supplies the heart, but not the arteries of the body. These nerves contain the entirely different chemical substance, acetylcholine. These nerve endings supply mainly the sinus node (pacemaker) of the heart and the heart's conduction system. During nervous stimulation, release of this substance causes the opposite effect of epinephrine and norepinephrine: slowing of the heart rate.

These special sets of nerves to the heart containing norepinephrine and acetylcholine, and the nerves to the arteries containing norepinephrine, are connected to the brain via the spinal cord, and in various normal situations they are stimulated to release the appropriate substance within the heart. Thus, the body has its own built-in mechanism for regulating both the rate and the strength of the heart's contraction, as well as the blood pressure. For example, a higher heart rate and more forceful contraction with activation of this "involuntary" nervous system, coupled with epinephrine release during exercise, enables the heart to increase greatly its output of blood and thereby meet the need of the rapidly working muscles of the limbs for extra oxygen. This involuntary (or "autonomic") nervous system also operates reflexly to control the action of the heart and the blood pressure. Mechanisms exist in the nervous system which "sense" when the blood pressure becomes too high, and *fewer* nerve impulses are sent to the norepinephrine-containing nerve endings (leading to a less forceful and slower heart beat, and relaxation of the small arteries), while *more* nervous impulses reach the acetylcholine-containing nerves to the heart (leading to an even slower heart rate). Together, all these effects tend to regulate the elevated blood pressure toward normal. Conversely, when the blood pressure becomes too low (such as in severe bleeding or shock), or even when a healthy individual suddenly stands up and the blood pressure drops, the body sends *more* nervous impulses through the nerves containing norepinephrine. The heart then beats more rapidly and forcefully, and contraction of the small arteries tends to increase the resistance to blood flow. These effects act to restore the blood pressure toward normal. These nervous reflexes controlling the heart and circulation operate on a moment-to-moment basis, helping to maintain the blood pressure at a relatively even level throughout the day.

Effects on the heart and blood pressure also are produced when the physician injects adrenalin or norepinephrine, since these agents can then reach the heart and small arteries by way of the bloodstream. Sometimes these agents are given by injection in order to stimulate the heart and circulation and to raise the blood pressure when there is circulatory collapse due to heart disease or other causes. Acetylcholine is rarely given to slow the heart rate because it is rapidly destroyed in the body and has many other actions, but a drug that *blocks* the effects of acetylcholine, atropine, is sometimes given to temporarily speed up the heart rate when it is too slow.

STARLING'S LAW OF THE HEART

How does the heart deliver the same amount of blood from the right ventricle as from the left? Obviously, if the amount of blood flow delivered from one ventricle were larger than from the other, the lungs or the systemic circulation would rapidly become flooded with extra blood. The atria and the two ventricles are able to pump at exactly the same number of beats per minute in synchronized fashion because of the heart's electrical conduction system, as alluded to above, but in addition there is a remarkable mechanism built into the heart muscle itself. This mechanism has been called "Starling's law of the heart" (described by the English physiologist, Ernest Starling in 1914). In simplest terms, this law states that the heart pumps out with each beat precisely that amount of blood which fills it prior to the contraction. If more blood is delivered, more is pumped out. The property of heart muscle responsible for the phenomenon is this: When any muscle is stretched while it is in the resting state, the number of chemical sites on the protein filaments that can come into contact is increased; the muscle will then contract more forcefully if it is stimulated electrically to contract (see Figure 2-5). Thus, if the right ventricle temporarily increases its output of blood, as it does for example during the transfusion of blood into a vein, the extra volume of blood passes through the lungs with several heartbeats, reaches the left heart and causes an increased stretch of the left ventricle during its filling phase. This increased stretch causes the left ventricle to contract more forcefully and so to eject the extra volume of blood. By this mechanism, the two separate pumps which compose the heart are kept in remarkably perfect balance minute by minute, and throughout the day.

Of course, certain diseases may affect only one side of the heart. For example, when the left ventricle is damaged by a heart attack, blood may back up into the lungs behind the failing left ventricle and cause lung congestion. In fact, a variety of disorders can produce failure of either the right or left pumping chambers (see Chapter 9).

REFERENCES

General

Selzer, A., *The Heart. Its Function in Health and Disease*, University of California Press, Berkeley, 1966.
You and Your Heart (E. M. 508), American Heart Association, New York, 1970 (pamphlet).

Scientific Works

Braunwald, E., Ross, J. Jr., and Sonnenblick, E. H., *Mechanisms of Contraction of the Normal and Failing Heart*, 2d ed., Little, Brown and Company, Boston, 1975.
Katz, A. M., and Brady, A. J., "Mechanical and Biochemical Correlates of Cardiac Contraction," *Modern Concepts in Cardiovascular Disease*, **40**:39, 1971.

Diagnosing Heart Disease

If heart disease of significance is suspected by the physician, either because of symptoms, an abnormal finding on physical examination, or a laboratory test, a series of other diagnostic studies may be undertaken. In addition to examination of the heart itself (feeling with fingertips the chestwall overlying the heart to search for abnormal pulsations or vibrations and enlargement of the heart; listening for abnormal heart sounds and vibrations with the stethoscope), other special studies may include the following:

1   *X-rays* of the chest, often with different views of all surfaces of the heart to search for enlargement of various chambers.

2   An *electrocardiogram* (EKG), sometimes supplemented by an exercise test, or by a three-dimensional electrocardiogram (vectorcardiogram).

3 A *phonocardiogram,* taken with a device which amplifies normal and abnormal sounds within each heartbeat and records them on moving strip charts.

4 An *echocardiogram*, which registers a "picture" of various moving structures within the heart by recording the reflected echoes from an ultrasound beam.

5 Measurement of the blood lipids (fats), consisting of *triglyceride* and *cholesterol* levels, which can be useful for detecting and managing some types of hardening of the arteries (atherosclerosis), as discussed in Chapter 7.

6 In some instances, highly specialized studies termed "cardiac catheterization" and "angiocardiography" may be indicated.

Since these procedures can assume great importance in the modern diagnosis of heart disease, each is considered in somewhat more detail below.

THE PHYSICAL EXAMINATION

By placing your right hand over the front of the chest beneath the breast at the left lower side, and then leaning far forward, it is usually possible to feel the normal heartbeat. When the heart is enlarged (as frequently is the case in the presence of heart disease), the physician often can ascertain which chamber of the heart is enlarged and also feel the abnormal movements and vibrations which may accompany heart disease. Upon listening to the heart with the stethoscope, physicians normally hear a sound when the two valves separating the pumping and receiving chambers (the mitral and tricuspid valves) suddenly close at the beginning of the pumping cycle, and they hear a pair of snapping noises as the two valves separating the pumping chambers from the arteries (aortic and pulmonic valves) snap shut at the end of each pumping cycle (see Figure 2-1). Each heart cycle therefore is accompanied by "lub-dup" sounds as these two sets of valves close in sequence, and it is followed by a pause before the next beat. As might be expected, in the presence of disease of these valves such closure sounds may be abnormally soft or loud. Other thudding sounds (termed "gallops") also sometimes are heard. Such extra thudding sounds in children and teenagers frequently have no significance, but in older patients may signify disease of the heart muscle.

What is Heart "Murmur"?   A sustained vibration (murmur) may be produced within the heart and can be likened to the noise of water as it rushes through a garden hose. Soft murmurs sometimes are heard in the normal heart. These so-called functional murmurs are particularly common in children and young adults, and they probably result simply from rapid circulation of blood across the normal heart valves. If one partially obstructs a garden hose, or if the faucet is opened more fully, the rushing sound becomes louder. In the same way murmurs result from turbulence in the blood as it rapidly passes through an abnormal heart valve as, for example, when a valve is narrowed by disease. The heart must then force a small stream of blood across the valve at high velocity in order to provide sufficient blood flow to sustain the body, and a loud murmur may be heard with the stethoscope.

To understand how the physician is able to interpret heart murmurs, it is necessary to know only two bits of information:

1   Murmurs, which originate in the four different valves of the heart, are heard at four different *locations* on the chest wall.
2   The *timing* of each murmur within the heartbeat tells whether the involved valve is narrowed or leaking.

Let us examine each of these statements more closely. Localizing the murmur to one of the valves is simply a matter of knowing where the heart lies in relation to the ribs (the "first" rib is just under the collarbone). For example, murmurs of the aortic valve are heard over the upper right chest (at the second rib) and those of the mitral valve are heard over the lower left chest (near the fifth rib). If one then recalls the function of each of the four heart valves, it can be predicted which phase of the heart's cycle will be occupied by a murmur when the valve is narrowed (termed "stenosis") and which phase when it is leaking (termed "insufficiency" or "regurgitation"). Again, to use the aortic valve as an example, since this valve separates the main blood vessel (aorta) leading from the left pumping chamber, it must be open as the pumping chamber contracts to eject blood and a murmur heard when this valve is narrowed (aortic stenosis) occurs *during* the contraction phase of the ventricles (Figure 5-2*B*). It therefore occurs simultaneously with the pulse in the arteries. The aortic valve closes when the pumping chamber (ventricle) relaxes in order to prevent blood from flowing backward from the aorta into the left ventricle, and therefore when this valve is leaking the murmur is heard *between* each contraction or pulse (Figure 5-2*A*). The timing sequence is exactly the opposite with the valves that separate the receiving chambers from the pumping chambers. For example, narrowing of the mitral valve (mitral stenosis) also produces a murmur during the resting or filling phase of the heart cycle, that is, between each contraction, but the murmur is heard in a different location on the chest wall from the murmur of a leaking aortic valve.

Some of the early records of heart examinations are interesting. Jean Nicholas Courvisart (1775–1821), one of Napoleon's physicians, described some features of the narrowing of the mitral valve in 1806:

> There are certain signs which allow us to recognize the affection in question. Among these there is a certain thrill,* difficult to describe, perceptible when the hand is applied to the precordial region, a thrill which comes without doubt from the difficulty which the blood finds in passing through an orifice which is not large enough for the quantity of blood which it is supposed to let pass.

Later, in 1826, the great French physician R. T. H. Laennec (who is credited with inventing the stethoscope) added further information by describing the sound of the murmur (or bruit):

> This thrill was not continuous but came at regular intervals of equal length—it was not synchronous with the pulse beat, it appeared rather to alternate with the beat. This sensation was not solely of

---

*A "thrill" is a term used to describe the vibrations which may be felt with the fingertips on the chest wall when there is a very loud heart murmur.

the touch; it seemed also that the sense of hearing was concerned in it (and)—the cylinder (stethoscope) applied between the cartilages of the fifth and seventh ribs, produced a dull bruit, very strong and quite like the sound produced by a file rubbing on wood. This bruit was accompanied by a purring, heard by the ear, which was evidently the same as that felt by the hand.

Other unusual sounds also may be heard through the stethoscope. For example, when there is an infection of the sac around the heart (pericarditis), a to-and-fro rubbing noise may be heard as the heart moves against the rough, inflamed surface.

THE ELECTROCARDIOGRAM

As discussed in Chapter 1, a group of specialized pacemaker cells in the right-sided receiving chamber (atrium) of the heart regularly produces a series of electrical signals at a rate of 70 per minute. As each electrical impulse spreads out from the pacemaker cells, the muscle cells of the heart are affected by the arrival of the impulse and are "depolarized." That is, they temporarily lose their resting electrical charge, a process which stimulates the muscle cells of the heart to then contract. The impulse, which starts in the pacemaker cells (sinus node), travels first over the two receiving chambers (atria), enters a special area (AV node) that delays the impulse, and then spreads by way of the special electrical conducting system into the ventricles. There it spreads into the muscular walls of these pumping chambers, causing them to contract. Thus, the atria are stimulated to contract first, then the ventricles.

As it arrives at each heart chamber, the electrical activity reaches all the muscle cells of the chamber nearly simultaneously. It is the *sum* of all these individual cell impulses recorded from the surface of the body that makes up the electrocardiogram. Pairs of electrodes placed on the skin detect this change in electrical potential, and the signal is then amplified electronically and used to drive a pen up and down, inscribing the electrocardiogram on paper moving at a constant speed. These electrodes are so arranged that pairs of electrodes placed on the arms and legs "look" at different surfaces of the heart, and in addition several electrodes are placed around the front of the chest, close to the heart. Each of the latter electrodes also is one of a pair which "looks" at the front of the heart. The electronic system is so arranged that as the electrical impulse travels sequentially through the chambers of the heart *toward* one of the electrodes, an upward movement of the pen of the electrocardiograph machine occurs, and as the impulse moves *away* from that electrode, there is a downward deflection of the pen. Thus, a moving line is inscribed as the paper passes beneath the pen and records the electrical charge first from the atria and then the ventricles; several recordings are made using different pairs of electrodes to examine the different surfaces of the heart, and these tracings constitute the standard electrocardiogram.

As the atria depolarize, just prior to their contraction, a small deflection termed the "P wave" is recorded (Figure 3-1). There ensues a short pause without an electrical signal (the delay as the impulse traverses the AV node), which is followed by a large signal called the "QRS complex." The latter is generated as the ventricles depolarize just prior to their contraction. The QRS electrical signal is much larger than that from the atria (P wave) because there are many more muscle cells in the thick-walled ventricles than in the atria. Finally, as the muscle cells recover (repolarize) between contractions, another slower signal follows the QRS complex (the T wave) (Figure 3-1).

What Type of Information Is Contained in the Electrocardiogram?

1 *Heart rhythm.* Since the recording paper is moving at a known speed, the physician can determine from the electrocardiogram the beating rate of the atria and the ventricles. Normally, each P wave is followed by a QRS, a sequence that occurs about seventy times per minute when we are at rest. It can be determined from the EKG if the ventricles are not depolarized each time a P wave occurs (an abnormal situation) and whether or not the impulse is following the normal conducting pathway to reach the ventricles. As will be discussed in Chapter 6, diseases which affect any part of the pacemaker or the conduction system of the heart can cause serious problems by interfering with the

THE ELECTROCARDIOGRAM

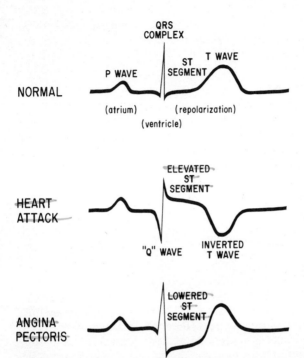

Figure 3-1 Examples of electrocardiographic tracings. The normal tracing records first electrical activity from the atrium (the P wave) and then activity (electrical depolarization) from the pumping chambers or ventricles (the QRS complex). The ST segment and the T wave reflect electrical repolarization of the ventricles.

During a heart attack (the second tracing), the QRS complex shows evidence of damage to the muscular wall of the pumping chambers by the presence of a "Q" wave. In addition, muscle damage is indicated by characteristic elevations of the ST segment and inversion of the repolarization wave (the T wave).

During an episode of chest pain, or angina pectoris, typical transient changes in the electrocardiogram often occur. This is the same change that may be produced during a stress test such as the Master's two-step test or a treadmill exercise test. This change is an abnormality in the repolarization of the heart consisting of a lowering or depression of the ST segment and indicates temporary insufficiency of the blood supply to the muscle of the pumping chambers.

heart's regular rhythm, with the orderly sequence of contraction during each beat (P wave followed by QRS), or with the rate of beating of the various chambers.

2 *Size of the heart's chambers.* By the *amount* of voltage generated (that is, the height of the P and QRS signals), the electrocardiogram can indicate whether or not the various heart chambers are enlarged, that is, whether or not there is an abnormally increased number of muscle cells in one or the other heart chamber. Usually it can be ascertained *which* chamber is enlarged by using different pairs of electrodes that, because of their position, tend to "look" at, or be closer to, one or another of the heart's chambers. For example, using certain electrodes which are placed around the front of the chest near the heart, it can be determined if the left ventricle is enlarged. The QRS signals recorded near the left ventricle will then record a voltage that may be twice the height of the normal QRS complex at that location.

3 *Muscle damage.* From the configuration of the electrical signal, often it is possible to determine whether or not the heart muscle has been damaged. When one of the coronary arteries which supplies blood to the heart is blocked, that zone of heart muscle may die. Initially, the only changes that are seen in the electrocardiogram relate to the recovery (repolarization) phase of the electrocardiogram (the area on the electrocardiogram just before and including the T wave) (Figure 3-1). When the cells are injured (and therefore unable to restore their normal resting electrical potential), this portion of the electrocardiogram becomes deformed, the segment of the tracing following the QRS is displaced, and the T waves may be inverted (Figure 3-1). Hours or days later, when the area of muscle is completely dead, there is loss of all the voltage which would normally have been generated by the region of muscle involved. Thus, when a heart attack has occurred, an electrode placed on the chest near the damaged zone may record a large early downward deflection instead of the usual upright QRS complex (Figure 3-1). This occurs because the dead tissue leaves a "hole," an electrically silent area, from which the normal voltage is not generated. All these changes in the electrocardiogram may be useful to the physician in identifying the occurrence of a recent heart attack. The changes in the QRS complexes (initial downward wave or "Q wave") are useful in identifying the location of an area of damage, and although this abnormality sometimes disappears in the months and years after

recovery of the patient, often Q waves persist and indicate that a heart attack has occurred in the past. The changes in the T waves and the ST segment of the electrocardiogram are transient during an acute heart attack.

The Exercise Electrocardiogram

In patients who have narrowing of the coronary arteries, but who have not suffered a recent heart attack, abnormalities may be seen in the recovery phase of the electrocardiogram, but *only* when the heart is placed under stress. Therefore, an exercise test may be performed during which the patient walks up and down a set of steps or on a moving treadmill, in order to increase heart rate and to place some stress on the heart. This stress normally causes an increased blood flow to the heart muscle through the coronary arteries, and under these conditions the electrocardiogram may reveal an insufficiency of coronary blood flow if the coronary arteries are significantly narrowed. Thus, impaired blood flow through a diseased coronary artery may not provide adequate oxygen to meet the heart's increased rate of metabolism during the exercise. Under these circumstances, abnormalities are seen in the recovery (repolarization) phase of the electrocardiogram. The cells do not recover their resting electrical charge normally, and deformed T waves and displaced ST segments (the region between the QRS and T wave) may occur transiently during the exercise, or for a short time thereafter (Figure 3-1).

In some patients with severe coronary heart disease, such abnormalities may be evident on the ordinary electrocardiogram, even when the patient is at rest. Such changes also may appear temporarily if an electrocardiogram is recorded during an attack of chest pain.

THE PHONOCARDIOGRAM

Sometimes it may be difficult to discern the sequence of various abnormal sounds and murmurs using the stethoscope alone, and a phonocardiogram can prove helpful. With this device, the sounds generated from the heart are detected by means of a small crystal microphone which is applied to the skin of the chest at various locations directly over the heart. An electronic signal is generated from the noise detected by the crystal and amplified to drive a pen which "draws" the sounds, moving up and down to record high frequency vibrations of the heart murmurs on paper moving at a known speed. The phonocardiogram can be recorded on the same paper as the electrocardiogram, and the latter then indicates exactly when the chambers are depolarized to contract. Normal and abnormal opening and closing sounds of the heart valves can be recorded and analyzed with this device. In addition, other abnormal sounds can be detected and it can be readily determined what types of heart murmurs are present. The phonocardiogram may also be recorded together with the waves of the pulses in the veins or arteries in the neck (measured from the pressure change in a small suction cup applied to the skin of the neck), which can give additional information about the relation that various sounds and murmurs bear to the contraction and relaxation phases of the heartbeat.

THE ECHOCARDIOGRAM

When a small crystal, a sound transmitter and receiver, is placed on the skin over any part of the body, the reflected sound waves often can be used to generate "pictures" of the underlying organs. The beam used is "ultrasound," very high-frequency sound out of the audible range (over 10,000 cycles per second), a portion of which is reflected back to the crystal when it encounters a tissue which differs in density from the adjacent tissue. This instrument has proved useful in identifying abnormalities in a number of areas (such as the abdomen and brain), and it has greatly facilitated the "noninvasive" evaluation of certain forms of heart disease. Thus, the sound beam is reflected from the external surface of the heart when it is adjacent to the lung, from the interface between the heart muscle walls and the blood contents of the chamber, and also from valve leaflets moving within the blood pool inside the heart. When the reflected sound is displayed on an oscilloscope as motion over the course of several heart cycles, it is possible to "see" the moving walls of the heart, the valves, and the aorta and pulmonary artery walls. Also, for example, in patients with narrowing of the mitral valve (mitral stenosis), the normal opening motion of the valve is absent and replaced by limited movement which can be clearly seen on the echocardiogram. Since the speed with which the sound travels through the tissues is known, the distance from the chest wall to the various structures, and between the structures within the heart can be determined accurately, and therefore the size of the heart chambers and the amount of excursion of valve leaflets can be determined with reasonable accuracy. Many new improvements are taking place constantly in ultrasound instruments, such as the development of an array of multiple crystals which simultaneously record many echoes, and these new devices in the future promise to give even better dynamic "pictures" of normal and abnormal heart structures.

CARDIAC CATHETERIZATION AND ANGIOCARDIOGRAPHY

The fact that all the veins and arteries of the body ultimately connect to the heart suggests the possibility of gaining access to the heart through a blood vessel, but it was not until 1925 that a young German intern named Werner Forssman inserted a catheter (a small flexible tube) through his own arm vein and into the right-sided receiving chamber and took an x-ray picture of the catheter inside his heart. This virtuoso accomplishment was followed up later by Drs. André Cournand and Dickinson Richards in the late 1940s, who passed a catheter even further to the right ventricle and into the pulmonary artery in patients with heart disease. These then-daring accomplishments subsequently resulted in the award of a Nobel Prize in Medicine to these three individuals. The modern era of cardiac catheterization had begun.

The term "cardiac catheterization" means simply that a tube is passed into the chambers of the heart. Today the tube, or catheter, is a small, flexible plastic tube less than one-eighth inch in diameter. The catheter is constructed of material that is not penetrated well by x-rays and can therefore be readily seen on the x-ray–television screen. The catheter is inserted through a vein in

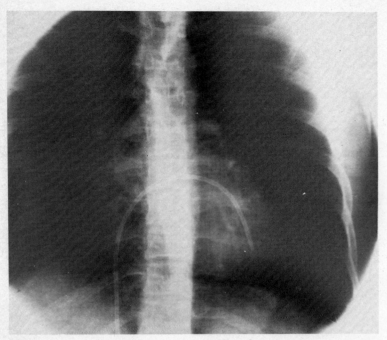

Figure 3-2 *Left panel:* X-ray taken during the course of a cardiac catheterization. The shadow of the heart can be discerned centrally within the chest, and the plastic catheter (white) (which is more opaque to the x-rays) is seen within one of the chambers of the heart. Through the catheter (tube), pressures can be measured and blood samples withdrawn.
Right panel: Angiocardiogram with injection of x-ray contrast liquid into left ventricle in a patient with leakage of the mitral valve (side view). The left pumping chamber, the aorta (arching vessel), and leakage of contrast material backward into the left atrium (small chamber beneath the aorta) can be seen. (Compare with Figure 5-1*B*.)

the arm or leg and observed on the screen as it is passed within the blood vessel toward and into the heart. The tube does not cause pain as its tip is passed through the blood vessels and heart, since their linings contain few nerve endings, and because the catheter is small and flexible it can be passed across the valves of the heart with little or no disturbance of the heart's function. Pressures can then be measured and injections or samples taken in the right-sided heart chambers (Figure 3-2, left panel).

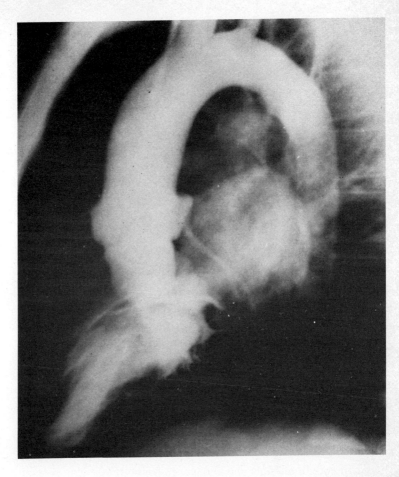

An important problem remained, however. Most serious
heart disease predominantly affects the *left*-sided valves and
heart chambers (coronary artery disease, for example, mostly
damages the left ventricle). Although it was possible to estimate
the pressure in the left-sided receiving chamber (left atrium) by
pushing the catheter tip far out into the lung and "wedging" it in a
small artery supplying the lung (a branch of the pulmonary
artery), the left side of the heart could not be reached directly.
This is because blood passing through the lungs must traverse

tiny capillaries, visible only under the microscope. Obviously, therefore, it was not possible to pass the catheter from the pulmonary artery through the lungs into the left heart chambers. During the mid 1950s, about 15 years after the first catheterization of the right heart, methods were finally developed for placing a catheter into the left-sided chambers of the heart.

Left-Heart Catheterization Numerous difficult and ingenious techniques were initially tried, including passage of long needles through the back, directly through the front of the chest, and even through the windpipe to reach the left-sided receiving chamber, which lies against the branch of the windpipe leading to the left lung. Most of these techniques had some dangers and disadvantages. At the present time, the left side of the heart is most commonly entered by passing a catheter into an artery in the arm or leg backward, or retrograde (against the flow of blood), up to the aortic valve and then across the aortic valve (while it is open) into the left ventricle. Another technique, using an approach through a vein, also is sometimes used for certain types of studies. In 1957, one of the authors (J. R.) was in the process of performing a right-heart catheterization and attempting, by manipulating the catheter, to find and cross a small hole that sometimes exists from birth in the partition, or septum, that divides the two receiving chambers (the right and the left atrium). A visitor from Chile, Dr. Emilio Del Campo, who was watching the procedure said, "It would be nice if you could burn a hole in the normal wall and get into the left heart that way." I replied that maybe one could find a way, and sometime later in a series of experiments in animals and cadavers I found that it was possible to accomplish this by pushing out a tiny needle, sheathed within a catheter, that was placed against the wall separating the right and left atrial chambers. This procedure (called "transseptal left-heart catheterization") allows a catheter to then be passed over the needle into the left atrium and across the mitral valve into the left ventricle.

These approaches for entering the aorta and left side of the heart are of importance in evaluating patients under consideration for surgery on the mitral and aortic valves. Recently the simpler approach of passing the catheter retrograde up an artery has been widely used since it also allows direct evaluation of the coronary arteries, the first branches of the aorta (see below).

What Can Be Accomplished through the Cardiac Catheter?

1 The catheter (which is filled with fluid) allows the recording of pressures in each of the heart chambers and in the vessels leading to and from the heart. The pressure wave is transmitted from the catheter tip, which lies at the appropriate location within the heart, to an electronic transducer and is then recorded on a moving stripchart. For example, by passing the catheter across a diseased aortic valve, it is possible to measure a higher pressure in the pumping chamber than the aorta if the valve is abnormally narrow, and by calculating blood flow, the exact severity of the narrowing can be determined.

2 Blood samples can be drawn through the catheter. These are used in measuring the amount of blood the heart is pumping per minute, and also for determining the location of certain inborn heart defects. For example, when there is a hole in one of the dividing walls of septum within the heart, red blood from the left side of the heart may cross through the hole and mix with blue blood from the right side of the heart. If the hole is between the receiving chambers (see Chapter 10, Inborn Heart Disease), when the catheter is passed into the right atrium and a blood sample withdrawn, an abnormally high content of oxygen is found in the blood from the right atrium. If the hole is between the two ventricles (ventricular septal defect), a high oxygen content is found in the blood sample that is withdrawn from the right ventricle. This "shunt" of blood from the left side of the heart to the right can therefore be detected by cardiac catheterization and the amount of the abnormal flow can be calculated. In other types of inborn heart disease, however, the pressures on the right side of the heart may be higher than those on the left, and a shunt of blue blood to the left-sided chamber occurs.

Tiny amounts of special materials (usually dyes) can also be injected through the catheter and their dilution, sampled at another location, is used to measure the amount of blood flow through the heart.

3 Special liquids can be injected rapidly through the catheter to mix with the blood, while remaining impenetrable to x-rays.

Therefore when an x-ray is taken, the inside of the heart chambers and blood vessels, wherever blood containing the special liquid reaches, can be "seen" indirectly on the x-ray film. A series of such x-ray films can be taken rapidly using a mechanical x-ray film changer or, more often, x-ray motion pictures (sixty pictures per second) are taken, a procedure called "cineangiocardiography" (Figure 3-2, right panel).

Angiocardiography Normally, as the left ventricle contracts, the mitral valve snaps shut to prevent blood from leaking backward into the left atrium, but if the mitral valve is diseased and leaking (Figure 5-1B), when the special x-ray contrast liquid mentioned above is injected through a catheter directly into the left ventricle, it mixes with the blood and then leaks backward from the left ventricle into the left atrium. This event can be seen in the x-ray movie, and the severity of the leak can thereby be determined (Figure 3-2, right panel). The manner in which the muscular wall of the pumping chamber (left ventricle) moves also is evident on the motion picture, and whether or not its contraction is normal can be evaluated. Leakage of the aortic valve can be studied by injecting the special liquid into the aorta.

Marked deformities of the heart chambers, valves, or blood vessels can occur with inborn heart disease. For instance, the heart chambers may be reversed, or the pulmonary arteries to the lungs may actually originate from the aorta, rather than the right-sided pumping chamber. The development of angiocardiography, with its ability to make pictures of the heart's anatomy during life, has made possible the accurate diagnosis of complex heart defects.

Coronary Arteriography The tip of a catheter can be placed directly into the orifice of an individual blood vessel as it originates from the aorta almost anywhere in the body, and a small amount of special x-ray contrast liquid can then be injected directly into the blood vessel. This technique has previously been used to visualize the anatomy of the blood vessels supplying the kidney, the bowel, or the brain on the x-ray film, and it is now widely used also to study the small blood vessels that supply the heart and the coronary arteries. The brief injection of a small amount of the liquid directly into the opening of each coronary artery using a catheter passed into the aorta from the arm or leg is quite safe, and all the branches of these arteries can be seen on the x-ray film (Figure 3-3). Whether or not any of the arteries has been completely or partially blocked by arteriosclerosis can

Figure 3-3 X-ray pictures taken during coronary arteriography. This procedure is carried out during cardiac catheterization and involves injection of a liquid, which is opaque (white) to x-rays, directly into the opening of the coronary artery.
Panel A: Injection into the right coronary artery of a normal human subject (compare with Figure 2-3). The plastic tube, or catheter, filled with contrast can be identified at the upper part of the picture. The channel of the coronary artery itself is widely open, and the branches which supply the muscle of the pumping chambers can be seen.
Panel B: Coronary arteriogram in a patient with severe coronary atherosclerosis. By comparison with the normal coronary artery, it can be seen that several areas of narrowing are present, and at the white arrow the coronary is almost completely blocked by an atherosclerotic region (see text). However, a small blood vessel can be seen to branch from the upper portion of the coronary artery and to run downward, rejoining the artery below the area of severe narrowing. This vessel is termed a "collateral" artery and serves to help maintain blood flow around the narrowed zone.

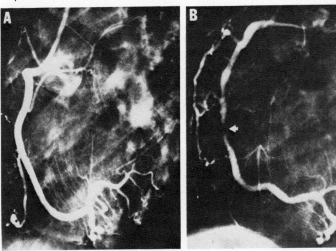

then be ascertained, and the amount of impairment, if any, of the muscular wall of the left ventricle can also be studied by an injection and motion-picture study of that chamber.

When are Cardiac Catheterization and Angiography Usually Done? At the present time, the major application of these methods is in the evaluation of patients with heart disease before considering a heart operation. Indeed, the great advances that have taken place in surgery of the heart would not have been possible without the development of cardiac catheterization and x-ray techniques for determining precisely the type of abnormality present and its severity. Certain congenital heart defects may be very complex, combining a number of different abnormalities. Some inborn defects presently are not correctable by operation, whereas others are readily repaired, and heart catheterization and angiocardiography must be employed to reach such decisions. In patients with valvular heart disease, catheterization may be carried out to determine how severely a valve is damaged, and whether or not more than one valve is involved. Coronary arteriography usually is performed to determine whether or not a blood vessel grafting ("coronary bypass") operation is feasible (Chapter 11) and where to locate the graft. Finally, sometimes cardiac catheterization is performed to determine whether or not a patient has significant heart disease at all. For example, some individuals have a heart murmur, or chest pain, that is shown by cardiac catheterization *not* to indicate the presence of heart disease, thereby relieving them of worries that sometimes develop into a "cardiac neurosis."

REFERENCES

General

How Doctors Diagnose Heart Disease, U.S. Department of Health, Education and Welfare, Public Health Service.

How the Doctor Examines Your Heart (E. M. 93), American Heart Association, New York, 1972 (pamphlet).

Scientific Works

O'Rourke, R. A., and Braunwald, E., "Physical Examination of the Heart," in *Harrison's Principles of Internal Medicine*, New York, McGraw-Hill, 7th ed., pp. 1075–1082.

Ross, J. Jr., "Cardiac Catheterization," in *Harrison's Principles of Internal Medicine*, New York, McGraw-Hill, 7th ed., pp. 1099–1106.

Ross, J. Jr., and O'Rourke, R. A., "Indirect Methods of Examination of the Heart," in *Harrison's Principles of Internal Medicine*, New York, McGraw-Hill, 7th ed., pp. 1092–1099.

Ross, J. Jr., O'Rourke, R. A., Peterson, K. L., Ludbrook, P., Crawford, M. H., Leopold, G. R., Karliner, J. S., Sobel, B. E., and Ashburn, W. L., "Non-invasive Methods for the Assessment of Cardiac Function," *California Medicine*, **119:**21, 1973. (Specialty Conference)

Role of General Factors in Cause, Prevention, and Treatment of Heart Disease

Before describing in some detail the various types of heart disease, it may be useful to consider first the magnitude of the problem and to discuss some general factors that appear to influence the occurrence and progression of heart disorders.

Diseases of the heart and circulation are the leading cause of death and disability in the United States, afflicting more than 27 million children and adults, and killing more than 1 million individuals annually. Among the 27 million people having heart and blood vessel diseases, high blood pressure is present in about 21 million, coronary heart disease and heart attack in over 4 million, rheumatic heart disease in 1.6 million, and stroke in 1.6 million. Cardiovascular diseases claim more lives than all other causes of death combined, and heart attack alone is the largest single cause of death in the United States, accounting for one-third of all male deaths between the ages of 35 and 65. Heart and blood vessel diseases cost the nation 19.5 billion dollars annually, including lost income and payments for medical care. In addition, cardiovascular diseases are responsible for the loss of approximately 62 million person-days of production each year. These data indicate the scope of the problem of heart and blood vessel diseases and make clear the need for prevention by reduction or elimination of factors which increase the risk of developing heart disease, and for the early diagnosis and treatment of established disease.

Atherosclerosis of the coronary arteries clearly is a major health problem, and the cause, effects, and specific treatment of this disorder are considered in detail in Chapter 7. It is worth pointing out here, however, that a number of environmental and other factors ("risk factors") greatly increase the likelihood that an individual will develop coronary artery disease. The established risk factors include high blood pressure, elevated blood lipids (cholesterol and/or triglycerides), excessive cigarette smoking, increasing age, and sugar intolerance (diabetes). Suspected risk factors include a sedentary life style, a family history of premature coronary artery disease, psychosocial tension, obesity, and a diet high in saturated fats and cholesterol.

OBESITY

Persons who weigh 20 pounds or more above their ideal body weight have an increased risk of both high blood pressure and coronary artery disease occurring together. If obesity occurs in conjunction with an elevated blood sugar, or a high serum cholesterol, it also significantly increases the risk of developing coronary heart disease. Thus, obesity itself may not be an *independent* risk factor, but it is importantly related to the development of coronary heart disease. Weight reduction often results in a decrease in blood pressure, improved sugar tolerance, and lower serum lipid levels, thereby reducing several of these known coronary risk factors. In patients who have experienced a heart attack, or who have coronary artery disease with chest pain, obesity has detrimental effects by placing an additional strain on the heart. Obesity can also increase symptoms in patients with valvular heart disease by increasing the workload of the heart.

DIETS

Low-cholesterol, Low-fat Diets The current epidemic of atherosclerosis has forced attention upon the nature of our diet. There is now considerable evidence that excessive ingestion of fatty foods can increase the blood fats or *lipids* (cholesterol and/or triglycerides) and that the "atherogenic diet" consumed by millions of Americans may be responsible in part for the finding that about 30 percent of American males over age thirty and under age forty-five have cholesterol levels in excess of 260 milligrams per 100 milliliters of plasma (mg percent). Although factors other than diet (such as sex, blood pressure, diabetes, genetic factors) also are important (see Chapter 7), the fact remains that the risk of developing coronary heart disease is about 3 times as great in men who have cholesterol levels above 260 milligrams per 100 milliliters as in men with levels under 180 milligrams per 100 milliliters. It is equally clear that weight reduction and diet can lower blood lipid levels.

What is this atherogenic diet? It consists mainly of eating hundreds of milligrams of cholesterol contained in meats, certain shellfish, and dairy products (one egg yolk alone contains about 300 mg of cholesterol!), and large quantities of fats, primarily of the saturated (animal) type rather than the polyunsaturated (vegetable or fish oil) variety. It is now well-established that in many individuals diets high in cholesterol and saturated fats can lead to elevated blood cholesterol levels. Diets high in carbohydrates can lead to increased blood triglyceride levels (mainly by stimulating triglyceride production in the body). Beef, lamb, and pork are particularly high in saturated fats and cholesterol; and eggs, shellfish, and organ meats (such as liver and sweetbreads) contribute greatly to a high intake of cholesterol. The increasing use of packaged foods, such as frankfurters and luncheon meats, has added to the high intake of saturated fats, and saturated-fat shortenings (lard) often are used in packaged bakery goods.

Concentrated sweets (soft drinks, candy, jams, frostings) and other carbohydrates, including alcohol, contribute to elevations of the triglycerides. It is of interest that today we eat about 3 times as much refined sugar as we did in 1850, with the average American now ingesting about 4 1/2 ounces of sugar daily.

The question of whether or not diminishing the blood lipids will prevent the development of atherosclerosis in young individuals, or reverse the disease when it is already established, is clearly an important one, and current evidence on this topic is discussed in Chapter 7. The answer is not yet available, but the circumstantial evidence that diet is important is sufficiently compelling to lead us to believe that a special diet should be used by individuals with elevated lipids, whether or not they have recognized coronary heart disease.

Recent research indicates that different patterns of lipid elevations in the bloodstream may require different types of treatment. Thus, a specific diet useful for one type of hyperlipidemia (high blood fats) may be inappropriate for another. These diets, and the medications that may be used in the treatment of these disorders, are discussed in Chapter 7.

"Special" Weight-reducing Diets   In recent years a large number of best-selling books have appeared on how to lose weight in a hurry. Unfortunately, many of these diets present special problems, and do not contain an adequate amount of all required nutrients.

One type of popular weight-reducing diet consists of severely restricting carbohydrate intake, while obtaining most of the daily calories from foods high in protein and fat. On such a diet, persons burn their own fat as a source of calories for energy, and weight loss is produced. However, this process produces acidic ketone bodies which, although they may depress the appetite, can also cause other problems, such as dehydration, elevated blood uric acid (sometimes with attacks of gout), or the development of kidney stones (see reference concerning the "ketogenic diet"). Moreover, such a high-fat diet can serve to increase blood cholesterol levels, particularly in individuals in whom these levels tend to be high on a normal diet. Finally, certain nutrients such as calcium and iron are deficient in this diet. For these reasons, an individual who wishes to reduce his weight should consult his physician before beginning a diet that requires severe carbohydrate restriction.

Other popular reducing diets with serious nutritional deficiencies include the "high protein–high water" diet, the "gelatin" diet, and the "skim milk and bananas" diet. These, and the low-carbohydrate diets mentioned above, are low in milk (calcium) and bread and cereal foods (thiamine, iron), and do not promote sound eating habits.* The Weight Watchers diet appears to supply low calorie intake with generally adequate nutrients and food variety.

Other "Fad" Diets   Many other diets have been proposed to correct supposed endocrine disorders, or to induce a desirable spiritual state, as well as to cause weight reduction.

The "hypoglycemic diet" is a low-carbohydrate, high-protein diet, frequently without calorie restriction, which is recommended by its advocates for relieving a variety of nonspecific symptoms (depression, chronic fatigue, allergies, etc.) which they attribute to a low blood sugar (hypoglycemia). In the great majority of instances, however, the blood-sugar level is not low, and such symptoms are not caused by hypoglycemia. The most common cause of a temporary low blood sugar is so-called reactive hypoglycemia, which occurs after a meal; this can occur in mild diabetics, for example. In most cases this does not require treatment, although occasionally, when it is troublesome, frequent feedings and a relatively low-carbohydrate, high-protein diet may be used. In some instances, injections of adrenal cortical extract (a hormone mixture obtained from the adrenal glands of domestic food animals) also are given "to increase the blood sugar," but they are of no value for this purpose. (An important statement on hypoglycemia in the *Journal of the American Medical Association* is listed in the references.)

---

*The compositions of a number of these diets are analyzed in detail in a booklet published by the California Dietetic Association: "A Dozen Diets for Better or Worse" (see references).

One diet popular for nearly twenty years consists of a 500-calorie diet plus injections of the hormone, human chorionic gonadotropin (HCG). However, claims for the use of HCG in the treatment of obesity have not been substantiated, and the diet does not provide an adequate range and quantity of nutrients.

A vegetarian diet provides adequate nutrition as long as it contains an adequate quantity of protein and essential amino acids. These can be obtained by adding skim milk, cottage cheese, and several eggs per week to the basic diet.

Low-Salt Diets   Patients with a persistently elevated blood pressure and patients with congestive heart failure usually require a diet that is low in sodium. In patients with high blood pressure, a reduction in the sodium intake is frequently associated with a reduction in the blood pressure, and some of the drugs which are successful for treating hypertension increase the excretion of salt (sodium chloride) and water by the kidneys. In patients with heart failure, the kidneys retain salt and water abnormally, leading to fluid accumulation in the lungs, in other organs such as the liver, and in the legs. In order to prevent this accumulation of fluid, it is necessary to limit the sodium intake. This is done by restricting the intake of foods rich in sodium, such as milk, bread, and soup, and by limiting the amount of salt used for seasoning. Salt substitutes, which contain little or no sodium, may be used as condiments to make the food palatable.

Vitamin E   Although vitamin E (tocopherol) deficiency in sheep, cattle, and rabbits may result in conspicuous abnormalities of the heart muscle, vitamin E deficiency in primates (apes, man) does not affect the heart even when other organs are involved. No heart disease in man has ever been clearly related to a vitamin E deficiency. The use of vitamin E in doses 10 to 50 times the daily requirement was recommmended nearly thirty years ago for the treatment of a variety of heart disorders, including angina pectoris, heart attack, and heart failure, but no convincing evidence of its effectiveness has been forthcoming in the intervening years.

EXERCISE

A number of studies have related the incidence and severity of coronary heart disease to differences in occupational activity. Men in sedentary occupations have been reported to have fatal heart attacks at a younger age than those whose occupations involved vigorous activity, and there is increasing evidence that regular physical activity may help prevent or delay the development of symptoms due to coronary artery disease. An occupational situation also could foster or diminish the development of coronary heart disease by altering a coronary risk factor, such as diet. However, comparative studies of population groups with similar dietary intake appear to show a greater incidence of coronary artery disease and heart attack in sedentary than in physically active workers. In a prospective study of 667 middle-aged London men, clinical symptoms of coronary heart disease (chest pain, heart attack) occurred more commonly among bus drivers than among the more-active conductors on double-deck buses; in another study, symptoms were more common among postal clerks, telephone operators, and executives than among the mail-carrying postmen. Although it is possible that no differences exist in the incidence of coronary artery narrowing by atherosclerosis in such studies, the incidence of clinical symptoms due to coronary artery disease in physically active individuals appears to be less than that for more sedentary persons.

Progressive exercise training may be of considerable benefit in preventing or delaying the onset of symptomatic coronary artery disease in normal individuals, and in reducing the severity of symptoms and mortality in patients who have clinical evidence of coronary artery disease. The question as to whether daily physical exercise results in the formation of new coronary arteries (collateral channels) in patients with coronary artery disease is unresolved. However, exercise training does reduce several of the risk factors which make an individual more prone to develop coronary artery disease, such as obesity and elevated blood lipids. Furthermore, the heart rate and blood pressure are reduced at any level of exercise in the well-trained individual, resulting in a decrease in the demands of heart muscle for oxygen at that degree of exertion. After a graded program of exercise training many patients with coronary heart disease show an improvement in angina pectoris, so that more exercise can be undertaken before chest pain develops.

Studies performed in Israel comparing the survival rate in patients with a prior heart attack who then underwent a program of progressive exercise rehabilitation, to that in similar patients who led a sedentary existence, showed a fivefold increase in mortality rate in the individuals who did not undergo daily physical exercise during a ten-year period of follow-up.

Currently there is considerable enthusiasm for daily exercise, such as walking, jogging, or swimming, as a measure in the prevention of symptomatic coronary artery disease. However, it is important to emphasize that exercise is not free of danger, both to the musculoskeletal and the cardiovascular systems. This is especially true for middle-aged individuals who may have unsuspected coronary artery disease, particularly those with coronary risk factors, and who suddenly undertake vigorous exercise after years of minimal physical activity. Such individuals should seek a physician's guidance before beginning a graded program of exercise training.

Exercise rehabilitation of patients with angina pectoris and/ or a previous heart attack is being recommended by many physicians. In several cities, cardiac rehabilitation centers have been organized where patients with known coronary artery disease are monitored for electrocardiographic changes, alterations in blood pressure, rhythm disorders, and symptoms during programs of progressively increasing exercise. Individualized exercise training programs at home are prescribed for each patient based on information obtained during this period of observed exercise. In many of these centers the patient undergoes electrocardiographic monitoring during his daily exercise, and he is retested at given time intervals, any change in his exercise program being related to his improved work performance.

However, the majority of patients with symptomatic coronary artery disease who undertake a period of exercise rehabilitation attempt to improve their exercise tolerance gradually, while under a physician's care, but not under direct supervision during exercise. Unfortunately, self-motivated exercise training generally has been less successful than formal, supervised exercise programs. Patients are cautioned to avoid sudden strenuous activity and to perform graded physical activity to an extent slightly less than that which brings on symptoms of chest pain, fatigue, or shortness of breath. Physical activity which produces slow progressive increases in heart rate, blood pressure, and cardiac output is less likely to produce symptoms than exercise which rapidly increases those factors which determine the oxygen demand of the heart muscle. For example, walking, jogging, swimming, and bicycling are less likely to produce chest pain than handball, volleyball, and tennis. Isometric exercise, such as sustained handgrip or lifting a heavy object, is to be avoided since this type of exertion is associated with a rapid increase in heart rate, blood pressure, and the oxygen demands of heart muscle.

Patients with coronary artery disease and symptoms should decrease their physical activity at high altitudes (greater than 6,000 feet), where the amount of oxygen in the blood is significantly reduced, and they also should decrease their degree of exertion in hot and humid environments because of the marked increase in heart rate which occurs with exercise under these conditions.

SMOKING

The nicotine contained in cigarettes causes an increase in heart rate and elevation of the blood pressure. Therefore, cigarette smoking increases the work of the heart and the demands of the heart muscle for oxygen. Also, the carbon monoxide in cigarette smoke combines with blood hemoglobin and reduces its capacity to carry oxygen. The consumption of twenty or more cigarettes daily is associated with a higher risk of having a heart attack (about three times that in nonsmokers). The risk of a heart attack is much less in pipe or cigar smokers, who generally inhale considerably less nicotine, but recent evidence indicates that the risk in these individuals is still greater than in nonsmokers. One must conclude that abstention from cigarettes can improve longevity in many individuals, although it is gratifying that the available data indicate that *former* cigarette smokers experience little if any added risk of coronary disease over nonsmokers. Thus, the danger does not appear to persist if the smoking is stopped. A direct cause-and-effect relationship between cigarette smoking and the presence of coronary artery disease has not been definitely established, but cigarette smoking (by increasing the heart's oxygen demands) increases the frequency of chest pain, heart attack, and sudden death in patients who already have coronary heart disease.

Various cardiac rhythm disturbances (particularly premature ventricular contractions) may be related to cigarette smoking, and the rhythm disorder may disappear when the patient gives up smoking. Rhythm disorders associated with cigarette smoking occur in patients with and without underlying heart disease; most likely they result from the stimulation of the sympathetic (involuntary) nervous system which follows nicotine inhalation.

SEXUAL ACTIVITY

There has been considerable apprehension regarding the effects of sexual activity on heart symptoms and function, particularly among patients with coronary artery disease. During intercourse there is an increase in the heart rate, a slight increase in blood pressure, and hyperventilation (rapid, deep breathing). This increase in heart rate and blood pressure is associated with an increase in the oxygen demands of the heart muscle, which may produce symptoms such as chest pain in patients with coronary artery disease. Occasionally fatal heart attacks have occurred during sexual activity; however, a recent research study has shown that the increase in heart muscle oxygen demands during sexual intercourse is mild, and may not impose as important a threat to patients with coronary artery disease as previously suspected. In a group of patients with at least one previous heart attack who were followed continuously by electrocardiogram, the average maximum heart rate attained during sexual activity was 117 beats per minute (range 90 to 144 beats per minute), and less than 20 percent of these patients with severe coronary artery disease had any symptoms of chest discomfort or palpitation. Moreover, the heart rate increase and the incidence of symptoms observed during sexual intercourse were no different from those occurring during other, normal daily activities.

In patients with mitral valve narrowing (stenosis) due to rheumatic heart disease, the symptoms of congestive heart failure may occur for the first time during sexual intercourse. The associated increase in heart rate, which diminishes the time available for emptying of the left atrium into the left ventricle, together with the increase in output of blood from the heart rapidly elevate the left atrial pressure resulting in the back up of blood in the pulmonary veins. This causes shortness of breath due to congestion of the lungs.

ALCOHOL AND THE HEART

In the past, physicians frequently prescribed small amounts of alcohol several times daily for patients with intermittent chest pain due to coronary artery disease, or with a previous heart attack. Any improvement in symptoms that occurs with this practice appears to be related mainly to the sedative effect of the alcohol, since it is now known that alcohol does not improve the coronary blood flow. Knowledge of the influence of alcohol on heart function has been expanded considerably in recent years by studies on the effects of acute and chronic alcohol use. It now appears that the acute administration of 2 to 3 ounces of alcohol consistently produces a transient reduction in heart function in subjects with and without heart disease.

In addition, rhythm disorders, heart failure, angina pectoris, and even sudden death have been associated with intoxication in patients with known cardiac disease. Some of these effects may be due to stimulation of the sympathetic nervous system by alcohol or one of its breakdown products.

Heart disease related to chronic alcoholism may be due either to associated nutritional deficiencies [e.g., thiamine (vitamin B_1)] or, more commonly, to severe disease primarily involving the heart muscle. On the basis of several clinical studies, it would appear that the cumulative effects of chronic alcohol intake can, without evidence of malnutrition, depress heart function and produce severe microscopic abnormalities of the heart muscle before clinical symptoms appear. Chronic alcoholics with heart muscle abnormalities may eventually develop symptoms of congestive heart failure and often have persistent heart rhythm disorders. Once symptoms of heart failure become apparent, the long-term outlook for survival is poor, and most patients with alcoholic heart muscle disease die within five years of the onset of symptoms.

In the mid 1960s, heart muscle disease associated with sudden severe heart failure and a 50 percent mortality was described among men drinking excessive quantities of beer. The "epidemic" incidence of this severe heart disorder in several cities coincided with the addition of cobalt sulfate to beer as a foaming agent. No further cases have occurred since cobalt was removed from the beer.

THE HEART OF THE ATHLETE

The trained, endurance athlete has been of interest to physicians and physiologists for many years. This attention has been prompted by the slow resting heart rate observed in the well-trained athlete, the frequent presence of partial heart block which disappears during exercise, the common occurrence of an "abnormal" electrocardiogram suggestive of coronary disease, and the frequent finding of an "enlarged" heart on chest x-ray. These observations initially led to a misunderstanding of the effects of athletic endeavors on the heart. Thus, strenuous exercise was considered deleterious, and was thought to cause heart enlargement similar to that seen in cardiac disease.

However, subsequent long-term clinical and physiologic studies of marathon runners, cyclists, and cross-country skiers have demonstrated no detrimental cardiac effects of endurance exercise. It is now apparent that the heart of the trained endurance athlete has an increased pumping capacity and is capable of providing more oxygen to body tissues at maximum work loads. There is no evidence that exhausting exercise imposes an ill effect on a healthy heart, nor is there any confirmation that strenuous athletic activity increases the risk of early death from cardiovascular disease.

EMOTIONAL STRESS

The association of such phenomena as palpitations, blushing, pallor, or fainting due to emotional stresses, and the increased occurrence of these symptoms in nervous or emotionally labile persons, have been well recognized. The obvious relation between emotion and cardiovascular function naturally has led to speculation and study of its possible role as causative or aggravating factor in diseases of the heart and blood vessels.

The fact that transient elevations of blood pressure can be produced by acute emotional stress and the observation that sustained hypertension often later develops in persons exhibiting such intermittently high blood pressures have suggested that emotional stress may play a role in the development of hypertension. However, a number of studies designed to demonstrate a correlation between the onset of hypertension and certain events in the life of the patient have so far been unrewarding.

Attempts to establish a relationship between emotional stress and coronary artery disease have been based on studies purporting to show a "coronary-prone personality;" that unusual life stresses exist in patients with coronary artery disease; that unusual emotional stresses precede an acute heart attack; or that elevations of blood cholesterol and triglyceride levels occur as a result of emotional stress. A number of studies have suggested that persons engaged in "stressful" occupations, such as physicians, dentists, lawyers, and accountants, have a high incidence of coronary heart disease.

Some authors have described a specific overt behavior pattern in association with clinical coronary artery disease, but others have failed to confirm these findings. Friedman describes a relationship between the so-called type A personality and an enhanced incidence of symptomatic coronary artery disease. These individuals have intense ambition, competitive drive, and a sense of urgency; they are constantly preoccupied with deadlines and make a sustained effort to achieve. He suggests that constitutional and personality factors also may influence the selection of an occupation, which then results in chronic socioeconomic pressure and emotional trauma.

The relationship of emotional stress to coronary artery disease (and indeed how to measure it) remains controversial, however, and some investigators have failed in their efforts to establish a definite association between executive responsibility, or various types of stressful industrial occupations, and the presence of known coronary artery disease.

Palpitation due to single or several premature beats, or to rapid cardiac rhythms, is among the most widely recognized symptoms of emotional stress, and for this reason emotional lability is commonly considered as a precipitating factor in many heart rhythm disorders.

Individuals under considerable emotional stress which may predispose to the development of symptoms when there is coronary artery disease, and patients with other cardiac disease in whom stress exacerbates their symptoms, should attempt to reduce stressful situations. The known physiologic effects of emotional stress, which are very similar to those of severe exercise, are sufficient to produce acute heart failure and occasionally prolonged chest pain in patients with advanced heart disease. Certain chronic situations such as family conflicts, unduly long work hours, boredom, unpleasant tasks, and fears of various sorts may create extremely stressful situations for the individual with heart disease, and often they can be modified. In many cases, a period of rest, a change of scene, an increase in social life, or a regular program of physical activity may be of great help in reducing such stress.

PREGNANCY

Heart disease is detected in approximately 2 percent of pregnant women in the United States. Usually such heart problems are due to valvular heart disease from previous rheumatic fever or to congenital defects. Other types of heart disease, such as coronary artery atherosclerosis or hypertension, occur less frequently in women of childbearing age.

During pregnancy there is an increase in output of blood from the heart in the mother, primarily due to an increase in heart rate, but also associated with some dilatation of the small resistance arteries of the body, blood flow through the placenta, and an increase in the total volume of blood in the circulation. This causes an increase in the workload of the heart, and, in patients with mild cardiac disease, symptoms may occur for the first time during pregnancy. Patients with more severe cardiac disease may receive treatment with a period of complete bedrest, as well as digitalis and diuretics. Even patients with serious heart disease usually can be treated successfully with medications, and only rarely is heart surgery during pregnancy necessary, or early delivery of the child required.

Patients with moderate or severe heart disease are strongly advised not to become pregnant, and adequate contraceptive measures should be taken. Interruption of pregnancy (therapeutic abortion) in women with heart disease is performed before the twelfth week of pregnancy for maximum safety and almost never after the sixteenth week of pregnancy.

Effects of German Measles and Drugs   Approximately 6 per 1,000 infants are born with structural malformations of the heart or great vessels. More than 25,000 infants are born annually with heart defects in the United States, but death from this cause has been reduced to less than 8,000 per year as advances in diagnosis and surgical treatment continue to make inroads on this serious problem.

Some heart defects and other birth malformations can be prevented by protecting women against rubella (German measles) during the first three months of pregnancy. A national immunization program has been established to prevent rubella in preschool and young school children, with whom the mother is in daily contact, and who usually are carriers of this disease. Although rubella is relatively mild as a children's disease, it can be extremely dangerous to the embryo, and immunization should spare many babies from inborn heart defects that result from rubella infection during the formative months in the womb.

The effects of drugs, cigarette smoking, high altitude, and radiation on the embryo formation during pregnancy are under study. In the early 1960s a new drug, thalidomide, was introduced as a supposedly harmless sleeping pill. This agent subsequently was found to cause a high incidence of birth defects, including major limb deformities and congenital heart disease. Thalidomide was rapidly removed from the drug market by the Federal Drug Administration.

DRUG ABUSE

The use of cannabis (marijuana) has greatly increased in recent years. Several studies have evaluated the cardiovascular effects of marijuana smoking in normal volunteer subjects. A significant increase in heart rate occurs in individuals smoking marijuana to up to twice the normal rate, and the increment in heart rate appears to be dose-related. A mild increase in blood pressure also is observed following the inhalation of marijuana. In some persons, frequent extra beats (ventricular in origin) occur after marijuana smoking. These increases in heart rate and blood pressure, and the occasional occurrence of premature ventricular beats, are most likely due to stimulation of the sympathetic (involuntary) nervous system, in a manner resembling that following the inhalation of nicotine.

The growing use of heroin throughout the United States has led to an increased incidence of bacterial infections involving the heart valves. The use of nonsterile syringes, needles, and filtering materials for the intravenous administration of heroin is associated with the introduction of bacteria into the venous system. These bacteria may then infect the valves, particularly of the right side of the heart, resulting in valve leakage and sometimes abcesses in the lungs. Bacterial infection in heroin addicts may also involve the left sides (mitral and aortic valves), producing severe valve leakage, congestive heart failure, and often death.

The use of amphetamines (such as Dexedrine for weight reduction or to keep awake and Neo-Synephrine in nose drops to reduce nasal congestion) stimulates the central nervous system, often producing an increase in heart rate and blood pressure. Large doses of amphetamines may precipitate heart failure in patients with underlying heart disease and often produce rhythm disorders in persons with normal or abnormal hearts.

REFERENCES

General

American Heart Association Cookbook, David McKay, New York, 1973.

A Dozen Diets for Better or for Worse, Foreword by R. B. Alfin Slater, School of Public Health, U.C.L.A.

How to Stop Smoking (E. M. 487), American Heart Association, New York, 1970 (pamphlet).

1973 Heart Facts (E. M. 509A), American Heart Association, New York, 1973 (pamphlet).

Stead, E., and Warren, G., *Low-Fat Cookery*, McGraw-Hill, New York, 1975.

Warshaw, L. J., *The Heart in Industry*, Harper and Row, Hoeber, New York, 1960.

The Way to a Man's Heart (E. M. 455), American Heart Association, New York, 1968 (pamphlet).

Zohman, L. R., and Tobis, J. S., *Cardiac Rehabilitation*, Grune & Stratton, New York, 1970.

Scientific Works

Aronow, W. S., and Cassidy, J., "Effect of Marihuana and Placebo-Marihuana Smoking on Angina Pectoris," *New England Journal of Medicine,* **291:**65, 1974.

Burch, G. E., and Giles, T. D., "The Burden of a Hot and Humid Environment on the Heart," *Modern Concepts in Cardiovascular Disease,* **39:**115, 1970.

"A Critique of Low-Carbohydrate Ketogenic Weight Reduction Regimens," *Journal of the American Medical Association,* **224:**1415, 1973.

Fox, S. M., Naughton, J. P., and Gorman, P. A., "Physical Activity in Cardiovascular Health," *Modern Concepts in Cardiovascular Disease,* **41:**13, 1972.

Mitchell, J. H., and Cohen, L. S., "Alcohol and the Heart," *Modern Concepts in Cardiovascular Disease*, **39**:109, 1970.

"Statement on Hypoglycemia," *Journal of the American Medical Association*, **222**:591, 1973.

Chapter 5

Diseases of the Heart Valves

The relative number of new cases of heart valve disease appears to be slowly decreasing, largely because of better control of rheumatic fever, which is the major cause of damaged heart valves. Improved control of rheumatic heart disease has resulted largely from the discovery that acute rheumatic fever follows streptococcal infections and that it can be prevented by treating this infection with antibiotics. Nevertheless, rheumatic valvular heart disease is present in over 100,000 children and 1.5 million adults in the United States, and it is responsible for about 15,000 deaths each year in subjects under sixty-five years of age. Less common causes of abnormal heart valves include congenital, or inborn, defects and faulty valve function resulting from infection or from heart attack, which can sometimes injure the attachments of the valves to the heart wall.

Rheumatic Fever

Deformities of one or more of the heart's valves most commonly are produced by the slow scarring process which follows acute rheumatic fever. This illness generally occurs in childhood, with the joint rheumatism as well as the damage to the heart valves following a particular kind of streptococcal infection of the throat or ears that is due to the Group A beta-hemolytic streptococcus. This same streptococcus also can cause the skin rash which constitutes scarlet fever. The episode of rheumatic fever is not a *direct* result of the bacterial infection; rather, it occurs in only a few patients, and it follows the "strep throat" by two or three weeks. Indeed, acute rheumatic fever occurs in less than 1 percent of individuals who have a streptococcal infection, and less than half of those who develop acute rheumatic fever subsequently develop chronic rheumatic valvular disease.

Rheumatic fever is a type of allergic inflammation in reaction to the foreign proteins (antigens) of the streptococcal bacteria; the defense proteins (antibodies) produced by the body then react not only with the streptococcus but also in an abnormal way to damage certain tissues of the body, most commonly the joints, heart muscle and heart valves, the brain, and the kidney. When the kidney alone is involved, an inflammation called "acute glomerulonephritis" occurs. With acute rheumatic fever, it is mainly the joints, heart, and brain that are affected. The major damage to the heart from rheumatic fever results from gradual scarring of the heart valves which occurs in the wake of the acute inflammation and may take years to become evident. Often this damage is enhanced by recurrent episodes of streptococcal sore throat followed again by rheumatic fever. Then, in late childhood or early adult life, the symptoms of valve damage ultimately appear.

Typically, the symptoms of acute rheumatic fever consist of swelling and redness of one or more joints (often several joints in succession), sometimes a skin rash, together with several weeks of fever. In some patients involvement of the brain results in peculiar, involuntary movements of the body which at one time were called "Saint Vitus' dance." Inflammation of the heart muscle also occurs during the acute illness, and disorders of the electrical system may be seen. Sometimes a bout of rheumatic fever in childhood goes unrecognized, and later the patient may only recall being told that he had "growing pains" (pains in the joints) or St. Vitus' dance. Recurrent attacks of acute rheumatic fever, which lead to progressive valve and heart muscle damage, can be prevented effectively by protecting against streptococcal infections with daily sulfadiazine or penicillin tablets. Sometimes a monthly injection of penicillin is given instead. Such preventive treatment may be continued throughout the life of the patient who has had an attack of rheumatic fever. In any individual, regardless of whether or not rheumatic fever has occurred previously, an acute streptococcal infection should be treated for 10 days with penicillin or other appropriate antibiotics in order to prevent the development of glomerulonephritis or acute rheumatic fever.

Effects of Valvular Damage

Normally, the delicate valve leaflets open and close each time the heart contracts. The valve scarring which results from rheumatic fever may take place over months and years, but eventually it causes the leaflets and their attachments to become thickened, adherent, and immobile. The involved valve may become narrowed ("stenotic"), leaky ("regurgitant"), or both. Mild damage to a valve may cause little or no difficulty, but when severe, it produces an inefficient pumping action of the heart. When a valve leaks, for example, a portion of the heart's energy is wasted in pumping extra blood backward and forward within the heart, and a certain volume of blood never passes out of the heart to reach the tissues. Eventually, as the damage progresses, the flow of blood out of the heart to the tissues becomes reduced, and the first symptoms of valvular disease may occur with exertion when there is inadequate delivery of blood and oxygen to the exercising muscles. Narrowing of a left-sided heart valve (mitral or aortic valve) can cause a build-up of back pressure in the blood vessels leading from the lungs. Thus, just as when a garden hose is partially compressed, pressure builds up behind the site of constriction. Shortness of breath may then result from stiffening of the lungs (which increases the work of breathing); later, leakage of fluid into the lung tissue, or actually into the air sacs themselves (with coughing up of fluid), may be caused by the high pressure, which further increases the difficulty in breathing. This sequence sometimes is sudden and severe, leading to "pulmonary edema," a frightening occurrence in which the patient almost drowns in his own secretions. Finally, longstanding overwork of the heart in patients with valvular disease eventually results in failure of the heart muscle itself, a condition which is described in more detail in Chapter 9.

The physician usually can determine the type of valvular damage on physical examination, since the sounds or murmurs produced by blood as it passes through a particular valve that is narrowed or leaking can be heard with the stethoscope. Sometimes, however, in order to determine precisely the severity of the damage to one or more valves, to assess whether or not the heart muscle is damaged, or whether the coronary arteries also are diseased, a cardiac catheterization test is carried out. Such a test often is undertaken when consideration is being given to a heart operation. The two most important valves in the heart, and unfortunately the two most often affected by disease processes, are those guarding the entrance and exit to the left-sided pumping chamber (the left ventricle); these are the mitral and aortic valves.

Narrowing of the Mitral Valve (Mitral Stenosis)

The mitral valve opens during the resting phase of the heart's cycle to allow blood to enter the left ventricle from the left-sided receiving chamber (the left atrium), and when the ventricle contracts to eject blood it closes to prevent backward flow of blood. Figure 5-1A illustrates narrowing of the mitral valve. The forward flow of blood across the valve is impeded, and pressure builds up in the left atrium in order to drive the blood across the narrowed orifice. Thus, a "pressure-gradient," or pressure difference can be measured across the valve. The high pressure in the left atrium is transmitted backward to the lungs through the pulmonary veins, and leakage of fluid into the lungs may take place. Eventually, the back pressure is transmitted all the way through the lungs to the pulmonary artery and right-sided pumping chamber (Figure 1-1), and in patients with severe and longstanding mitral stenosis, the muscle of the right-sided pumping

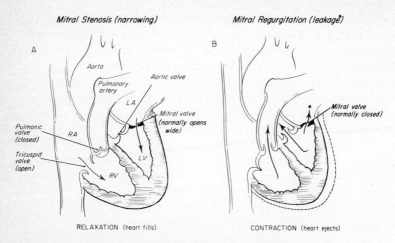

Figure 5-1 Diagram showing the effects of disease of the mitral valve. In both panels A and B the diseased mitral valve is shown in black.

Panel A: With narrowing of the mitral valve (mitral stenosis) caused by scarring, the valve is unable to open widely as it normally does (illustrated by the normal tricuspid valve on the right side of the heart). Therefore, during the relaxation phase of the heart cycle, a high pressure develops in the left-sided receiving chamber (the left atrium, LA) and the rate of blood flow forward into the left ventricle is reduced.

Panel B: With leakage of the mitral valve due to scarring (mitral regurgitation) the mitral valve fails to close normally (as does the normal tricuspid valve on the right side) and blood is not only ejected forward into the aorta but also backward into the left-sided receiving chamber each time the heart contracts. This results in excessive work of the heart and an inefficient contraction.

chamber may fail. This, in turn, leads to high pressure in the veins of the body (visible on the back of the hands and in the neck) and leakage of fluid (edema), which causes swelling of the ankles or abdomen.

Other complications of mitral stenosis are quite common. When the left atrium carries a high back pressure and its wall becomes stretched, the normal passage of the electrical impulse through the atrial wall may become impeded. Under these conditions, patients may develop a rapid, disorganized, and ineffective contraction of the atrium termed "atrial fibrillation"

(Chapter 6). This disorder is not fatal, since the atria serve only as booster pumps, but it may lead to an even higher pressure behind the narrowed mitral valve and increased symptoms. This complication also occurs late in the course of other valvular lesions, and occasionally in otherwise normal individuals.

Sometimes (most frequently in patients with abnormal heart rhythms) blood clots develop in the enlarged left atrium of patients with mitral stenosis. This occurs primarily because of the sluggish blood flow in that chamber resulting from the narrowed valve. Pieces of the adherent blood clot then occasionally may break loose (an "embolus"), and be carried out in the arterial bloodstream to the aorta and thence to the head, the kidneys, legs, or other organs. If such blood clots are sizable, they can block the blood flow through an artery and result in stroke (brain damage) or damage to other organs, as discussed below.

Leakage of the Mitral Valve (Mitral Insufficiency or Regurgitation)

Normally the mitral valve closes to prevent backflow of blood when the left ventricle contracts, but when the valve does not close completely, part of the blood goes backward with each heartbeat (Figure 5-1B). Therefore, the left ventricle must pump more blood than normal, and some of its effort is wasted. The extra volume of blood is passed back into the left atrium with each beat, and if the leak is large, eventually it causes the pressure to rise in that chamber, just as in patients with mitral stenosis. In addition, the left ventricle eventually grows very large and its muscle may fail due to the long-standing overwork. In patients with moderate mitral regurgitation the only symptom may be fatigue, due to somewhat reduced pumping action of the heart, but when the leakage is very severe, shortness of breath and failure of the right heart occur as with mitral stenosis.

Narrowing of the Aortic Valve (Aortic Stenosis)

The aortic valve normally opens wide during contraction of the left-sided pumping chamber (left ventricle) to allow the ejection of blood into the aorta. When the aortic valve is narrowed (Figure 5-2B), the left ventricle has difficulty in ejecting blood across the

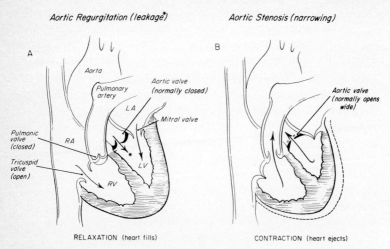

Figure 5-2 Diagram showing the effects of disease of the aortic valve. In both panels the diseased aortic valve is represented in black. In *Panel A*, which illustrates the effect of aortic regurgitation or leakage, the aortic valve on the left side of the heart normally behaves like the pulmonic valve on the right side. However, when the aortic valve is scarred and unable to close properly, blood leaks backward from the aorta into the left-sided pumping chamber (LV) while the heart is relaxed and filling from the receiving chamber. This results in loss of pressure in the aorta during the rest phase of the heart cycle and excessive blood flow into the left ventricle because of the leakage, causing increased work of that chamber. *Panel B* shows the effect of narrowing of the aortic valve (aortic stenosis). Normally, the aortic valve opens wide during heart contraction (like the normal pulmonic valve shown). However, when it is narrowed and scarred, a high pressure is built up in the left-sided pumping chamber in order to force blood across the narrowed valve opening. This causes increased work of the left-sided pumping chamber.

narrowed orifice and therefore must develop a high pressure during its contracting phase. To use the garden hose analogy again, the development of this high pressure allows the pumping chamber to overcome the resistance of the narrowed opening. With each heartbeat, therefore, a large pressure gradient across the valve exists (as with the narrowing of the mitral valve), and in order to maintain a satisfactory blood pressure in the aorta (100 to 110 millimeters of mercury) the ventricle must develop a pressure of 200 or 250 millimeters of mercury during its ejecting phase. With time, the left ventricle tends to develop a greatly thickened muscular wall, and patients with aortic stenosis tend to faint easily and to develop pain in the chest due to inability to supply enough oxygen to the overworked and greatly thickened heart muscle. As with the other types of valvular disease, failure of the heart muscle eventually occurs due to overwork of the muscle of the left ventricle.

Leakage of the Aortic Valve (Aortic Regurgitation or Insufficiency)

The aortic valve normally closes during the resting phase of the heart's cycle to prevent blood from passing backward from the aorta into the left ventricle while the ventricle is at rest and filling from the atrium. With leakage of the aortic valve, some of the blood that was pumped forward in the previous heartbeat leaks back into the left ventricle (Figure 5-2A). The ventricle is now filling from two directions, and it must then deliver forward an extra amount of blood, as well as the normal quantity. Under these circumstances, the volume of blood delivered with each heartbeat may be 2 or 3 times the normal amount, leading to a very striking accentuation of the arterial pulses. As with leakage of the mitral valve, this wasted effort results eventually in failure of the heart muscle.

Right-Sided Valve Disease

The tricuspid valve, which guards the entrance to the right ventricle, is rather uncommonly damaged by rheumatic fever, but when narrowing or leakage occur, they resemble these lesions at the mitral valve. Usually, this valve is involved only when the aortic or mitral valves also are diseased. Sometimes, high back pressure behind a narrowed or leaking tricuspid valve causes swelling of the ankles and other difficulties.

Significant disease of the pulmonic valve is very infrequent in rheumatic heart disease, although deformities of this valve as well as the tricuspid valve are common with inborn heart disease.

The Medical Treatment of Valvular Heart Disease

Heart surgery for valvular heart disease, in which valves are repaired or replaced with either an artificial valve prosthesis or a grafted tissue valve, is discussed in Chapter 11. When the disease of the valves is moderate, or when symptoms are mild, surgical treatment may not be recommended, and management with medications to strengthen the heart muscle, together with a low-salt diet or diuretic agents to eliminate the extra salt and water that tend to be retained in the presence of heart disease (see Digitalis and Diuretics, Chapter 9) may maintain the heart patient in comfortable condition for many years. In the individual who has had one attack of rheumatic fever, of course, the most important thing that can be done to limit development of valvular heart disease is to prevent the recurrence of streptococcal throat infections by means of a prophylactic antibiotic given continuously, as discussed above.

Other measures include careful attention to diet, weight reduction, and avoidance of overly strenuous exertion. Patients with recognized valvular heart disease are also usually advised to take antibiotics in high dosage immediately before and after dental extractions, root canal work, or even mechanical cleaning, after various surgical procedures, and during childbirth. This precaution is taken because damaged valves are susceptible to infection by the transient swarm of bacteria that are released into the bloodstream at these times. Infection on a diseased mitral or aortic valve ("bacterial endocarditis") can cause severe further damage and may be difficult to cure. Recently, with the increased use of addictive drugs such as heroin by intravenous injection ("mainline"), often using unclean syringes and containers, infections of normal as well as diseased heart valves, and particularly those in the right side of the heart, have been reported with increasing frequency.

Atrial fibrillation, a rapid disorganized electrical activity of the receiving chambers (atria), quite frequently occurs in valvular heart disease. Digitalis usually is employed to slow the response of the ventricles to this rapid beating of the receiving chambers. Digitalis also is used to increase the strength of the pumping chambers when the muscle fails. Both of these problems are discussed in more detail in subsequent chapters.

Blood Clots

The development of blood clots within the left atrium tends to occur particularly in patients with mitral stenosis and atrial fibrillation. (The ineffective, rapid beating of that chamber tends to slow blood flow through it and lead to formation of clots on its walls.) When such clots repeatedly break loose to form floating emboli in patients with mitral stenosis, surgery on the heart may be indicated. However, when the valve narrowing is not sufficiently severe to warrant operation, clot formation can be controlled by the use of "blood-thinning" agents (anticoagulants). One such agent (Coumadin) interferes with synthesis by the liver of protein-clotting factors which normally circulate in the blood. This medication must be taken daily and results in reduced normal clotting of the blood. When these drugs are used, it is necessary to check the degree to which the blood clotting is inhibited by periodic blood samples so that the blood does not become too "thin" and bleeding occur. These drugs are the same as those used to prevent clotting (sometimes called "thrombosis" or "thrombophlebitis") in the veins of the legs, a condition which can lead to the breaking loose of clots which may then travel to the lung, as discussed in an earlier chapter. When attention is directed to proper dosage and to blood tests every few weeks, these agents are effective and can be used for many years. They also may be used to prevent clot formation on artificial heart valves.

If, despite adequate treatment with various drugs, salt restriction, and other general measures, disabling symptoms persist and the valvular disease is severe, surgical treatment usually is recommended.

REFERENCES

General

1973 Heart Facts, (E. M. 509A), American Heart Association, New York, 1973 (pamphlet).

Selzer, A., *The Heart. Its Function in Health and Disease*, University of California Press, Berkeley, 1966.

Scientific Works

Rackley, C. E., and Hood, W. P., "Quantitative Angiographic Evaluation and Pathophysiologic Mechanisms in Valvular Heart Disease," *Progress in Cardiovascular Disease*, **15:**427, 1973.

Reichek, N., Shelburne, J. C., and Perloff, J. K., "Clinical Aspects of Rheumatic Valvular Disease," *Progress in Cardiovascular Disease*, **15**:491, 1973.

Ross, J. Jr., "Acquired Valvular Heart Disease," in *Textbook of Medicine*, Paul B. Beeson and Walsh McDermott, (eds.), W. B. Saunders Company, Philadelphia, 14th ed., 1975.

White, P. D. and Donovan, H., *Hearts. Their Long Follow-up*, W. B. Saunders Company, Philadelphia, 1967.

Chapter 6

Diseases of the Electrical System: Heart Rhythm Disorders and Heart Block

The most common complaint of individuals with a heart rhythm disturbance is an unpleasant awareness of the heartbeat, of "skipped beats," or a fluttering in the chest (sometimes called "palpitations"). Others have no such sensations despite marked electrical disorders. Sometimes symptoms develop as a secondary effect of the abnormal rhythm on heart function. For example, a patient with coronary artery disease may develop chest pain during a bout of sudden, rapid heart action. In this situation, the sudden increase in heart rate increases the oxygen usage of the heart, and the diseased coronary arteries are unable to deliver the needed extra coronary blood flow. Inadequate output of blood from the heart may result from a sudden, very slow heartbeat such as occurs in "heart block." In this condition, blood flow to the brain can be insufficient to maintain cerebral function, and a clinical syndrome results which is characterized by sudden transient loss of consciousness or convulsions. This condition is commonly called "Adams-Stokes attacks" after two nineteenth-century Irish physicians, but is more properly termed the "Morgagni-Adams-Stokes syndrome" after the Italian physician-pathologist who in 1761 initially described the relation between convulsions, or epileptic seizures, and a very slow pulse.

During the past few years, many advances have taken place in our understanding of the heart's electrical system and in the development of special forms of treatment. The use in coronary care units of electronic monitoring systems for continuously recording the electrocardiogram and thereby detecting abnormal rhythms, and the monitoring of patients outside the hospital by means of continuously recording the electrocardiogram on port-able magnetic tape recorders, has made it possible to detect electrical disorders that were never before recognized. The purposeful use of a brief electrical discharge ("countershock") applied to the outside of the chest to treat dangerous, rapid cardiac rhythms and rapidly revert them to normal, and the use of surgically implanted electronic pacemakers to maintain a normal heart rate in patients with very slow rates, have constituted major advances in the treatment of these potentially fatal heart rhythm disturbances. In addition, new medications have been developed for the treatment of abnormal cardiac rhythms which are more effective and less toxic than those previously available.

Basically, rhythm disorders of the heart (sometimes called "arrhythmias") are characterized by one of three findings: a changing interval between several heartbeats (irregular rhythm); interference with the passage of the electrical impulse through the heart's conduction system ("heart block"); or a heart rate that is faster or slower than the normal resting range of 60 to 100 beats per minute.

The normal pacemaker of the heart, the sinus node, is located in the right atrium. Its special electrically active cells form electrical impulses. The normal rate of impulse generation (seventy per mimute) can be influenced by various physiologic stimuli (such as exercise), by hormones and drugs, as well as by pathologic processes. Each impulse leaves the sinus node and transverses the receiving chamber or atrium to reach the atrio-ventricular (AV) node, a small collection of specialized conducting cells situated in the lower portion of the atrium; there, the impulse is delayed for less than one-tenth of a second (Figure 2-2). The electrical impulse then travels down a special conduction pathway analogous to a "wire" (the common bundle), which in turn divides into a right bundle branch and a left bundle branch. These two bundles spread out along the inner surfaces of the right and left pumping chambers (ventricles). The end-branches of this electrical conducting system are formed by special cells located within the muscle of the ventricles, the so-called Purkinje cells (after a nineteenth-century Czechoslovakian microscopist). These cells are concerned primarily with conduction of the electrical impulses directly to the heart muscle. Thus, electrical impulses normally pass through the two bundle branches and the Purkinje cells to reach the working muscle cells of the ventricles.

All the cells of the heart have the ability to maintain an electrical potential across their cell walls. However, all cells do not have the property of automatic activity, which is responsible for the normal spontaneous rhythm of the sinus node, for certain "protective" or "escape" rhythms, and for some rhythm disorders. Cells which possess this potential for automatic activity are located principally in the sinus node, but also in the AV node, the conducting bundles, and in Purkinje cells. Only these special cells, and not the muscle cells themselves, are capable of "firing" automatically.

The rate of impulse formation in automatic cells varies with the physiologic state of the individual subject, and it is also governed by the properties of the type of cell itself. Although the normal rate of electric impulse formation in the sinus node is sixty to one hundred impulses per minute, physiologic variations or severe stresses may drive the sinus rate as low as forty or as high as two hundred beats per minute (see Figure 2-6). Should the sinus node pacemaker cells for some reason diminish their rate of impulse formation to a sufficient degree, automatic cells in the AV node will take over control of the heart at a slower rate of forty to sixty impulses per minute. Should the AV node also fail to function, pacemaker cells (Purkinje cells) in the ventricles will then "escape" and take over, but they will drive the heart at an even slower rate—twenty to forty impulses per minute. This normal decreasing rate of impulse formation at different locations from the sinus node down to the Purkinje cells in the ventricles provides a safety mechanism whereby electrical pacing centers of the heart farther down the conduction pathway can take over should the normal center fail. Normally, however, the lower (and slower) pacemakers do not initiate such function as long as a pacemaker with a higher rate is driving the heart.

EXTRA BEATS

Any heartbeat that arises in a location outside the normal sinus pacemaker and occurs earlier than the next expected beat is called a "premature beat." Premature beats often arise in the atria, less commonly in the AV node, and frequently in the Purkinje cells of the ventricles. Such premature beats are often the precursors of continuous rapid atrial, nodal, or ventricular rhythms, particularly when such premature beats occur very frequently (more than ten per minute).

Atrial extra beats (Figure 6-1) are seen in individuals of all ages, and often they occur in the absence of heart disease. However, disease of the atrial muscle predisposes to such premature beats. Emotion, fatigue, excessive alcohol use, tobacco, and coffee all may cause atrial premature beats in normal individuals. Such beats also may result when the atrium becomes overfilled and stretched (as often occurs in congestive heart failure or rheumatic heart disease), when there is drug intoxication (such as digitalis excess), or when lack of oxygen supply affects the atrial muscle (coronary heart disease). Such impulses, as well as premature beats originating in the AV node, can be easily recognized on the electrocardiogram because they use the heart's normal conducting pathway to reach the ventricles, and the QRS complex from the ventricles is therefore normal (see Figure 3-1).

Ventricular extra beats are the most common form of rhythm disturbance, both in normal subjects and in patients with heart disease. Such premature beats, which start in the ventricle

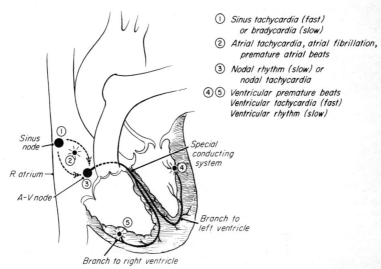

Rhythm Disorders

① Sinus tachycardia (fast)
   or bradycardia (slow)
② Atrial tachycardia, atrial fibrillation,
   premature atrial beats
③ Nodal rhythm (slow) or
   nodal tachycardia
④⑤ Ventricular premature beats
   Ventricular tachycardia (fast)
   Ventricular rhythm (slow)

Sinus node
R. atrium
A-V node
Special conducting system
Branch to left ventricle
Branch to right ventricle

Figure 6-1 Diagram showing the most common electrical disturbances of the heart's *rhythm*. The numbers and stars indicate the various locations in which such rhythm disorders can arise. For description see text.

(Figure 6-1), spread through the heart in a backward direction, through the muscle rather than the special conducting system, and therefore they produce a large, usually wide QRS complex which is readily recognized on the electrocardiogram. In some persons who are apparently normal, such premature beats may persist for many years without ill effects. However, they also may be caused by all types of heart disease, and sometimes they result from an excessive digitalis dosage. Ventricular extra beats also commonly occur in patients with heart failure, and they are present temporarily in the great majority of patients who suffer a heart attack. They may result as well from a low blood potassium level, from the use of coffee (caffeine), tobacco, or alcohol, and from many of the drugs which stimulate the sympathetic nervous system (such as the amphetamines—"pep pills"). An inadequate blood oxygen level in patients with severe lung disease predispos-

es to ventricular premature beats. Exercise may precipitate
ventricular premature beats, even in some normal subjects.

The Treatment of Extra Beats Therapy is indicated when
they produce disturbing palpitations, chest pain, or shortness of
breath, when they occur in patients with known heart disease, or
when they are considered likely to lead to abnormal, rapid atrial
or ventricular rhythms. In normal subjects who have palpitations
due to frequent premature beats, the cessation of cigarette
smoking, limiting coffee ingestion, or reducing excessive alcohol
intake may result in disappearance of the extra beats. In some
normal subjects, the use of medications such as quinidine or
procainamide, which suppress electrical impulse formation in
abnormal locations (but not the sinus node), is necessary to
prevent disturbing symptoms from premature atrial and ventricular beats.

In patients with an acute heart attack, ventricular premature
beats often precede a serious and sustained ventricular rhythm
disorder. For this reason, lidocaine, a medication given by
intravenous injection which eliminates extra beats without disturbing heart function, often is given to such patients whenever
ventricular premature beats are observed during continuous
monitoring of the electrocardiogram in the coronary care unit.

RAPID HEART RHYTHMS

A heart rate over 100 beats per minute (called a "tachycardia")
may originate in the sinus node, in an abnormal location in the
atrium, in the AV node, or in the Purkinje cells within the
ventricles. Although the range of the sinus node rate is normally
set at 60 to 100 beats per minute when we are *at rest*, this does not
mean that all heart rates outside this range are abnormal.

Rapid Sinus Rate (Sinus Tachycardia) A heart rate greater
than 100 beats per minute is occasionally found in normal
subjects at rest without evidence of cardiac disease; moreover,
heart rates induced by exercise or emotional stress in the adult
often are in the range of 100 to 150 beats per minute, and

sometimes are as high as 200 per minute if the exercise is severe. Sinus node rates over 100 normally are present in infants and young children.

A rapid rate of the sinus node can result from medications such as atropine and some of its derivatives (which frequently are used as gastrointestinal antispasmodics and for certain eye troubles). Also, inhalant medications used for asthma, thyroid extract, as well as the social use of "drugs" such as alcohol, nicotine (in tobacco), caffeine (in coffee), and marijuana all can increase heart rate.

Abnormally rapid sinus node rates also can occur in association with generalized disease states. Fever is the most common cause, but anemia, heart failure, excessive secretion of thyroid hormone by an overactive thyroid gland (called "hyper-thyroidism" or "thyrotoxicosis"), severe bleeding, and infections each can cause a rapid sinus rate.

No specific treatment is usually necessary for this type of rapid heart rhythm originating in the normal sinus pacemaker other than discontinuing medication or drugs when they are the cause, or treating the underlying disease which is producing the rapid heart rate.

Rapid Regular Atrial Rhythm (Atrial Tachycardia) Rapid cardiac rhythms which originate from abnormal sites in the atrium outside the sinus node (Figure 6-1) or in the AV node (but not in the ventricles) are sometimes called "supraventricular tachycardia." They are fairly common both in normal subjects and in patients with heart disease. This type of abnormal rhythm is rapid and regular, the heart rate usually being 160 to 200 beats per minute, and it is often a recurrent problem. Usually it begins and ends very abruptly ("paroxysmal atrial tachycardia"). It is rarely complicated by difficulties such as heart failure or low blood pressure. Individuals having this type of rapid rhythm may experience it very infrequently (once or twice a year), or it may occur often and be quite troublesome.

This disorder also occurs in patients who have a rather rare, abnormal conduction pathway between the atria and the ventricles which allows the electrical impulse to easily bypass the AV node, which normally slows down the impulse. The electrocardiogram is often very abnormal between attacks and indicates to the physician the existence of this abnormal pathway (called the "Wolff-Parkinson-White syndrome," one of whose discoverers was the late Paul Dudley White). Treatment for this condition is often difficult, and occasionally the abnormal pathway has to be divided surgically.

The treatment of the usual type of rapid, abnormal atrial rhythm is variable. Maneuvers which produce slowing of the heart rate, such as applying pressure and rubbing the fingers over the carotid artery in the neck near the jaw ("carotid sinus stimulation"), or the induction of nausea are often effective in terminating the rapid rhythm. The use of digitalis also frequently is effective in the treatment and prevention of this disorder. In some patients, medications such as quinidine, which suppress extra impulse formation, are required. Quinidine and another drug, procainamide, act to suppress sites of abnormal electrical impulse formation and therefore are frequently useful in prevention as well as in the treatment of extra beats and rapid atrial and ventricular rhythms. The administration of propranolol, a medication which blocks certain effects of the involuntary nervous system (and the effects of epinephrine, which speeds up the heart rate and the conduction of impulses through the heart), also may be effective.

Atrial fibrillation is a cardiac rhythm in which there are very rapid, ineffective, and irregular atrial contractions at a rate of 400 to 600 per minute (Figure 6-1). The beating of the ventricles also becomes irregular, but fortunately their rate is much slower than that of the atria. The rate of the ventricles is dependent on how many of the electrical impulses from the atrium are able to pass through the AV node, which normally slows the sinus impulse, but it may be as high as 180 or 200 per minute. Atrial fibrillation is a common disorder and may be either sustained or intermittent. Occasionally, it is found in apparently healthy persons. However, much more commonly it occurs in patients with heart disease, and it frequently complicates rheumatic valvular disease, coronary artery disease, hypertension, or hyperthyroidism. The sudden onset of atrial fibrillation in the patient with heart disease may precipitate failure of the heart.

Digitalis, which decreases the number of atrial impulses that are conducted through the AV node, is used in patients with chronic atrial fibrillation to slow the rate of the ventricles. In patients with atrial fibrillation in whom the ventricular rate has been slowed by digitalis, the addition of quinidine may be successful in the restoration of regular sinus rhythm. Electric countershock (see below) is an alternative and often more successful method of reverting atrial fibrillation to normal rhythm. Patients whose atrial fibrillation has been reverted to sinus rhythm usually continue to receive digitalis and quinidine indefinitely, in order to prevent subsequent episodes of atrial fibrillation. Often, however, in chronic heart disease the atrial fibrillation becomes permanent.

Rapid, Regular Ventricular Rhythm (Ventricular Tachycardia) When several consecutive ventricular premature beats (Figure 6-1) occur at a rapid rate, over 120 beats per minute, ventricular tachycardia is present. The disorder may complicate any form of heart disease, but it occurs most commonly in patients with coronary artery disease, particularly those experiencing a heart attack. The rhythm is very rare in the normal heart.

When ventricular tachycardia is sustained, its effects are extremely detrimental to heart function, and the blood pressure usually falls. This rapid rhythm originates in the ventricles, in the Purkinje cells, and the poor heart function is a consequence not only of the rapid rate, but also of the backward, slow progression of the electrical impulse through the muscle of the ventricles, rather than via its normal route. The rapid heart rate further increases the demands of the diseased heart muscle for oxygen, and the output of blood from the heart diminishes. Ventricular tachycardia frequently deteriorates to ventricular fibrillation, an even more serious rhythm disturbance, which is very rapidly fatal if not treated promptly.

The treatment of ventricular tachycardia is the intravenous injection of lidocaine, which is particularly useful for abolishing this rhythm (and extra ventricular beats) in patients with acute heart attack. If the disorder persists, electric countershock is used.

Ventricular fibrillation is a very rapid, disordered series of electrical impulses originating in the ventricles. It is associated with completely ineffective heart pumping action, and hence there is no blood pressure, and rapid loss of consciousness and death ensue. It may follow an episode of ventricular tachycardia, or it may be initiated at once by a premature ventricular contraction which occurs close to the preceding beat. Death occurs within a few minutes after the onset of ventricular fibrillation unless the ventricle is "defibrillated" by electric countershock.

Another electrical problem which also occasionally causes circulatory collapse is *cardiac arrest*, in which no electrical activity of the heart is evident.

ELECTRIC COUNTERSHOCK

The sudden discharge of electrical current across the chest is used in the treatment of various heart rhythm disorders. This technique can be lifesaving in the emergency treatment of ventricular tachycardia and ventricular fibrillation. The brief flow of the electrical current (which is stored in a capacitor and discharged as direct current across the chest and hence the heart) causes no significant damage to heart tissue. However, the electric countershock briefly interrupts all abnormal impulse formation in the heart (it "depolarizes" all cells) and, after a short pause, the automatic sinus node then takes over and normal rhythm resumes.

Electric countershock also is performed on an elective basis, since it is often successful in changing chronic atrial fibrillation to sinus rhythm. The patient is usually put to sleep briefly with a short-acting anesthetic agent. The electrocardiogram is monitored continuously, and two lubricated paddles, with insulated handles to protect the operator, are placed on the patient's chest. A brief, short electric shock is then transmitted to the patient's chest. Very small currents often are effective with atrial rhythm disorders, and the whole procedure usually requires less than thirty minutes; complications are rare. Much larger electrical currents usually are needed to "defibrillate" the thick-walled ventricles.

SLOW HEART RHYTHMS

Slow Sinus Rate (Sinus Bradycardia)   A sinus node rate of less than sixty beats per minute is the most common type of slow heart rhythm, and it occurs in both normal subjects and patients with cardiac disease. It is particularly frequent in elderly patients, even in those with no sign of heart disease. Sinus bradycardia also is often found in well-trained athletes, especially those whose activities involve sustained effort, such as long-distance runners. It may develop in some individuals during sleep. A slow sinus rate also can result from drugs which slow the heart rate (such as morphine), from diminished thyroid function, and it accompanies a very low body temperature. Sinus bradycardia generally needs no treatment, unless the slow heart rate appears to predispose to premature ventricular contractions or other rhythm disorders, and occasionally it requires treatment in patients who have associated dizziness or fainting spells.

Heart Block   This is the most common abnormal cause of slow heart rate, and it may occur at any location within the heart: in the sinus node, the AV node, or in the electrical conduction system to the ventricles (Figure 6-2). If impulses fail to travel out of the sinus node, one or more heartbeats may be missed completely, and if this occurs regularly, the heart rate can be very slow. If no impulses at all emerge from the sinus node, a lower pacemaker such as the AV node usually "escapes" and initiates the heartbeat at a rate slower than the normal sinus rate. Such blocks in the sinus node are quite uncommon, however. A much more common cause of a slow heart rate is the occurrence of block somewhere in the conducting pathway between the atria and the ventricles (Figure 6-2). The block may exist in an incomplete form, in which there is an abnormally long delay in the transfer of the sinus impulse through the AV node and *some* of the impulses fail to be transmitted, or *complete* heart block may occur, in which none of the impulses from the sinus node or the AV node are transmitted to the ventricles. In the latter situation, an independent pacemaker in the ventricles becomes the automatic pacemaker and drives the heart, but at a very slow rate (often thirty or forty beats per minute). This disorder

Disorders of Electrical Conduction

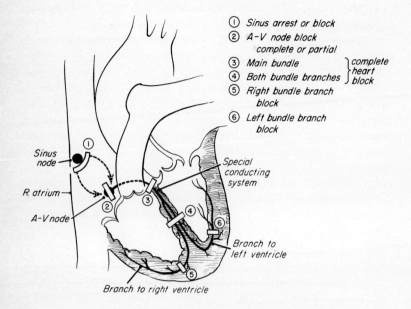

① Sinus arrest or block
② A-V node block
   complete or partial
③ Main bundle   ⎤ complete
④ Both bundle branches   ⎬ heart
⑤ Right bundle branch   ⎦ block
   block
⑥ Left bundle branch
   block

Sinus node

R. atrium

A-V node

Special conducting system

Branch to left ventricle

Branch to right ventricle

▭ – sites of potential complete or partial heart block resulting
in delayed or absent conduction of electrical impulses

Figure 6-2 Diagram showing sites of abnormal *blockade* of the heart's electrical conducting system. The white bars indicate where the most common types of block occur. For further discussion see text.

can be recognized on the electrocardiogram because the atrial electrical waves (P waves) are faster and have no relation to the slowly occurring widened QRS complexes from the ventricles (see Figure 3-1).

Complete heart block sometimes occurs as a congenital (inborn) abnormality, but more commonly it is due to heart disease acquired later in life. Complete heart block which is transient is particularly common in patients with an acute heart attack, and it also occurs in patients with chronic coronary artery disease or valvular heart disease. At first, the block may be intermittent and cause fainting or seizures (Adams-Stokes attacks, mentioned earlier) or it can become permanent; in many individuals with permanent or intermittent chronic complete heart block an electronic pacemaker may be required.

If one of the bundles of the conduction system to the right *or* the left ventricle fails to conduct the electrical impulse (Figure 6-2), a condition exists called *bundle branch block*. The electrocardiogram is abnormal and shows a wide QRS complex from the ventricles, but since most of the electrical conduction system from the atria to the ventricles is intact, the heart rate is normal and the electrical impulse simply spreads around the involved bundle branch to reach the pumping chamber. Of course, when *both* bundle branches fail to function, complete heart block results [just as when the AV node fails to transmit impulses, or the common bundle is blocked (Figure 6-2)].

ELECTRONIC PACEMAKERS

Surgeons discovered a number of years ago when operating on the human heart that if small electrodes were attached directly to the surface of the pumping chambers, artificially delivered electrical impulses from an electrical power source using quite small amounts of current could "pace" the heart at a normal rate. Usually, such a pacemaker is necessary because of complete heart block and the need to speed up the ventricles, which are beating at a very slow rate (perhaps forty per minute). Although electrodes can be directly implanted on the surface of the ventricles by means of an operation, the method now usually employed for artificially pacing the heart (either temporarily or permanently) is to place an electrode catheter, a long flexible tube which is passed through a vein in the neck or the arm, into the chamber of the right ventricle. The electrodes at the tip of the catheter are positioned against the inner wall of the ventricle and the electrical pacemaker impulse then drives the heart, its rate being higher than the patient's own rhythm. The energy source for the pacemaker catheter is a battery pack. For temporary pacing (as during a heart attack), the battery is outside the body and attached to one end of the catheter. A temporary pacemaker also is used to initiate the cardiac beat in patients with cardiac arrest. In patients who require a permanent pacemaker, the catheter is inserted via a small neck vein and left completely under the skin, the battery also being implanted under the skin of the chest or abdomen. Such pacemakers are used primarily in the treatment of slow rhythms, particularly in patients with incomplete or complete heart block, and drive the heart at about seventy beats per minute. "Demand" pacemakers function only when the patient's natural heart rate falls below a certain level.

The average life of a permanent pacemaker battery is two to three years, but considerable variability exists. In order to detect impending pacemaker battery failure, it is essential that patients with permanent pacemakers be evaluated on a routine basis and increasingly often during the second year following the pacemaker insertion. When one or more cells in the battery begins to fail, the number of pacemaker impulses per minute changes slightly from its preset rate. This change in pacemaker rate may be recognized from the electrocardiogram, or even more accurately by the use of an electronic-rate counter which measures the interval between pacemaker impulses to one-thousandth of a second. The pacemaker battery pack, located under the skin of the chest or abdomen, must be replaced by means of a small surgical procedure when the electrocardiogram shows evidence of pacemaker failure (skipping of paced beats), when changes in the pacemaker firing rate indicate impending battery failure, or when the time is reached at which pacemaker failure usually occurs. In some medical centers, the pacemaker battery is routinely changed at 24 months, even in patients who have not yet shown definite evidence of impending battery failure.

A recent advance in the care of patients with permanent pacemakers has been the development of "pacemaker centers" which receive telephone transmissions of the patient's electrocardiogram from the home. Electronic evaluation of pacemaker function is then carried out. Such facilities are particularly useful to elderly patients in whom frequent office or hospital visits are impractical and require considerable effort. The use of telephone transmission of the electrocardiogram enables the physician to evaluate pacemaker function at regular intervals more conveniently, thereby detecting impending battery failure more reliably and allowing implanted pacemaker batteries to be left in place longer (sometimes up to four years).

The relatively short life-span of such pacemaker batteries has led recently to the development of an atomic energy pacemaker, which is expected to last ten to twenty years. The use of atomic pacemakers is expensive and has so far been limited to animal experiments and to selected young patients.

Atropine, a drug which blocks involuntary nervous impulses which slow the heart, and isoproterenol, a medication which stimulates the heart rate, are sometimes used temporarily in patients with heart block. However, the majority of patients with complete block will require the insertion of a temporary or permanent intracardiac pacemaker.

REFERENCES

General

Living with Your Pacemaker (E. M. 516), American Heart Association, New York, 1971 (pamphlet).

Scientific Works

Fozzard, H. S., and Dasgupta, D. S., "Electrophysiology and the Electrocardiogram," *Modern Concepts of Cardiovascular Disease*, **45**:29, 1975.

James, T. N., "Changing Concepts in Electrocardiography," *Modern Concepts in Cardiovascular Disease*, **39**:129, 1970.

Keller, J. W., Gosselin, J. A., and Lister, J. W., "Engineering Aspects of Cardiac Pacemaking," *Progress in Cardiovascular Disease*, **14**:447, 1972.

Chapter 7

Diseases of the Coronary Arteries: Chest Pain and Heart Attack

Far and away the most common cause of serious heart trouble in the United States, and the leading cause of death, is disease of the coronary arteries. In fact, few individuals do *not* have a close friend or relative who has experienced or died from a heart attack. Coronary heart disease has assumed almost epidemic proportions in certain Western countries, and unfortunately, it has become relatively commonplace to hear of heart attacks occurring in individuals near age forty, or even younger. Heart attack alone was responsible for nearly 700,000 deaths per year in the United States in 1969, more than twice the number of deaths (320,000) attributed to the next leading cause, cancer. It is estimated that over 4 million Americans have coronary heart disease.

Coronary heart disease travels under a variety of names, and considerable confusion exists in most people's minds concerning its precise meaning. The terms "hardening of the arteries," "arteriosclerosis," or "atherosclerosis" are used to indicate a disease process which occurs in a specific set of blood vessels: the arteries of the systemic circulation (Figure 1-1); it almost never involves the veins of the body or the blood vessels to the lung. When the disease process involves the arteries supplying the brain, it can cause stroke; when it involves the arteries to the legs, it can cause pain (sometimes called "claudication"); and when it occurs in the coronary arteries, which supply the heart, it can cause chest pain ("angina pectoris") and heart attack. Atherosclerosis is characterized by a progressive buildup of fatty materials or lipids (triglycerides and cholesterol) within the walls of the arterial blood vessels. This process eventually leads to narrowing, or to actual blockage of the channel of the vessel involved.

The Cause of Coronary Artery Disease

In recent years many important facts have emerged, but the ultimate cause remains unknown. Clearly, the disease becomes more common with increasing age, and there is undoubtedly a long "silent period" while the fatty deposits gradually build up within the blood vessels. This view is supported by postmortem examinations made in young individuals, such as servicemen killed in Korea, which established that the arteries to various vital organs (particularly the heart) often showed moderate atherosclerosis. These individuals were, of course, at the time entirely without symptoms or other evidence of heart disease. It is now the opinion of many scientists that much of the lipid moves into the blood vessel walls directly from the bloodstream. Therefore the concentration of these fatty substances in the blood over a prolonged period of time may be of the utmost importance in producing the disease in susceptible individuals, and it seems logical that diet would be a significant factor. Some of the evidence relating blood levels of lipids and diet to coronary artery disease is the following:

1   The occurrence of coronary heart disease is unusual in world populations having low cholesterol and fat levels in the blood, and in most populations the disease incidence is directly related to the level of blood lipids.

2 The disease incidence is highest in countries such as Finland and the United States, where dairy and meat products rich in fat and cholesterol compose a relatively large portion of the diet. Moreover, when groups native to areas in which the consumption of these foods is low (such as the Orient) move to Western countries (and a "Western diet"), the incidence of coronary heart disease increases.

3 Factors other than diet which tend to increase the blood levels of fatty substances are associated with an increased likelihood that coronary artery disease will develop. For example, members of families with certain inborn or genetic errors of fat metabolism causing blood lipid values to be markedly elevated occasionally die even as teenagers from coronary heart disease. Also, women tend to develop coronary artery disease ten to twenty years later in life than men, a fact which may be related to the tendency of the female sex hormones to cause lower lipid levels in the blood.

4 Studies in animals have shown that diet-induced elevations of blood lipids can cause atherosclerosis in the coronary arteries and other blood vessels.

Although the incidence of coronary heart disease is higher in individuals with elevated blood lipids, and in populations on "Western diets," it should be emphasized that the disease occurs in some individuals in whom the blood levels of fats and cholesterol are normal. In addition, not all individuals with elevated blood lipids develop serious atherosclerosis. Therefore, it remains to be proven whether diet, faulty handling of fatty substances by the body's metabolism, hereditary factors, or all these are responsible for atherosclerosis. Nevertheless, while "guilt by association" does not constitute proof, there is enough evidence for an association between elevated blood lipids and coronary disease to warrant efforts to lower blood lipids when they are high through diet or drug treatment, as discussed further below.

Risk Factors

There are several factors which increase the likelihood that an individual will develop coronary heart disease. The proven risk factors are:

1   High blood pressure
2   Elevated blood lipids (cholesterol and/or triglycerides)
3   Excessive cigarette smoking
4   Diabetes
5   Age

The chances that a male having none of the first four will have a heart attack before he is age sixty-five are less than one in twenty, but if one factor is present, the risk increases twofold, and if two factors exist, his chances of having a heart attack by that age are about one in two, or 50 percent! Physical inactivity, obesity, and life stress also may increase the chances of having a heart attack, although these factors have not yet been proven to increase risk.

High blood pressure clearly accelerates atherosclerosis, and the risk of coronary heart disease is directly related to the level of blood pressure. Obesity is associated with an increased incidence of the disease, but this effect may be in part related to the positive relation between high blood pressure and obesity. Considerable information has been derived from a long-term study of the population of Framingham, Massachusetts, sponsored by the National Heart and Lung Institute. For example, some predictions from these studies concerning the "high risk individual" are as follows:

1   In males aged 30 to 49 who have a blood cholesterol level over 260 milligrams per 100 milliliters, over a 14-year period the incidence of coronary heart disease is about three times as great as when the level is less than 180 milligrams per 100 milliliters.
2   In males 45 years of age, if the systolic blood pressure is elevated to 160 millimeters of mercury and the cholesterol is over 260 milligrams per 100 milliliters, over a four-year period the incidence of coronary heart disease is about five times as great as when the systolic blood pressure is 110 millimeters of mercury and the cholesterol less than 180 milligrams per 100 milliliters.

Smoking is accompanied by an increased risk of heart attack—males who smoke one pack of cigarettes per day being twice as likely to have a heart attack as the nonsmoker. We shall discuss further these risk factors and what can be done to prevent coronary heart disease more fully at the end of this chapter (see also Chapter 4).

The Symptoms and Mechanism of Heart Pain (Angina Pectoris)

As described in Chapter 2, the coronary arteries bring oxygen-rich blood to the heart. When a deposit of fatty substance (cholesterol and fats) builds up within the wall of one of these vital arteries, the blood channel eventually may become critically narrowed (Figure 7-1). The first symptom from such an occurrence may be pain in the chest. Initially, the pain may occur only during severe exertion, or with marked emotional stress. At those times the blood pressure and the heart rate increase, enhancing the work of the heart and therefore augmenting its need for oxygen. Normally, the coronary arteries then open up more widely, thereby providing more blood to the heart to meet these needs. However, when an artery is narrowed, it becomes unable to widen further, and the region of heart muscle supplied by that artery receives insufficient oxygen. When this occurs, a pressure sensation, or squeezing pain behind the breastbone (angina pectoris), may be felt. Ordinarily, by promptly stopping the activity, the heart rate slows down, the increased work demands on the heart are relieved, and the pain disappears within one or two minutes. Although the zone of heart muscle supplied by the artery functions poorly and contracts only weakly during such brief episodes, no permanent damage to the muscle is produced (Figure 7-1). The exact mechanism behind the pain is unknown, but it may be related to the accumulation of chemical substances released by the heart muscle during oxygen lack, which then stimulate pain-sensitive nerve fibers within the heart muscle.

One of the earliest accurate descriptions of angina pectoris was that by the English physician William Heberden (1710–1801) in an account first published in 1768.*

But there is a disorder of the breast marked with strong and peculiar symptoms, considerable for the kind of danger belonging to it, and

*From Heberden, William: *Commentaries on the History and Cure of Diseases*, Boston, 1818.

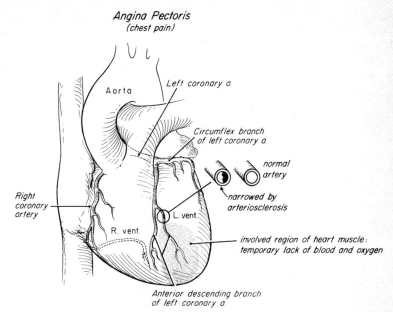

Angina Pectoris
(chest pain)

Figure 7-1 Diagram of the heart showing the coronary arteries and the pumping chambers, the right ventricle (R. vent.) and left ventricle (L. vent.). A branch of one coronary artery (coronary a.) is involved by atherosclerosis. The localized accumulation of lipid substances in the wall of the artery, which partially narrows a segment of the anterior descending artery, is indicated in black. When the demands of the heart for oxygen are increased (such as during exercise), an insufficient amount of blood reaches the region of heart muscle supplied by the involved coronary artery (stippled area). Temporarily, that region of muscle therefore contracts poorly and, in addition, chest pain ("angina pectoris") is experienced. The pain and temporary lack of oxygen are relieved when the exercise is stopped.

not extremely rare, which deserves to be mentioned more at length. The seat of it, and sense of strangling, and anxiety with which it is attended, may make it not improperly be called angina pectoris. They who are afflicted with it, are seized while they are walking, (more especially if it be uphill, and soon after eating) with a painful and most disagreeable sensation in the breast, which seems as if it would extinguish life, if it were to increase or continue; but the moment they stand still, all this uneasiness vanishes. In all other respects, the patients are, at the beginning of this disorder, perfectly well, and in particular have no shortness of breath. . . . The pain is sometimes situated in the upper part, sometimes in the middle, sometimes at the bottom of the os sterni, and often more inclined to the left than to the right side. It likewise very frequently extends from the breast to the middle of the left arm. The pulse is, at least sometimes, not disturbed by this pain, as I have had opportunities of observing by feeling the pulse during the paroxysm. Males are most liable to that disease, especially such as have passed their fiftieth year. After it has continued a year or more, it will not cease so instantaneously upon standing still; and it will come on not only when the persons are walking, but when they are lying down, especially if they lie on their left side, and oblige them to rise up out of their beds . . . . The termination of the angina pectoris is remarkable. For, if no accidents intervene, but the disease go on to its height, the patients all suddenly fall down, and perish almost immediately. . . .   The angina pectoris, as far as I have been able to investigate, belongs to the class of spasmodic, not inflammatory complaints, for:

In the 1st place, the access and the recess of the fit is sudden.
2dly, There are long intervals of perfect health.
3dly, Wine, and spirituous liquors, and opium afford considerable relief.
4thly, It is increased by disturbance of the mind.
5thly, It continues many years without any other injury to the health.
6thly, In the beginning it is not brought on by riding on horseback, or in a carriage, as is usual in diseases arising from scirrhus or inflammation.
7thly, During the fit the pulse is not quickened. . . .

With respect to the treatment of this complaint, I have little or nothing to advance: Nor indeed is it to be expected we should have made much progress in the cure of a disease, which has hitherto hardly had a place or a name in medical books.

Not long thereafter, in 1775, the Scottish anatomist John Hunter found in a postmortem examination of an individual dying after having had angina pectoris for several years that "the two coronary arteries from their origin to many of the ramifications of the heart were become one piece of bone." With observations such as these, the modern understanding of this disorder began.

The Symptoms and Mechanism of a Heart Attack (Myocardial Infarction)

As diagramed in Figure 7-2, eventually the fatty deposit may become of sufficient size to completely block the coronary artery; sometimes a blood clot forms at the site of a fatty deposit in the blood vessel wall. Occasionally, the narrowing becomes so severe that even without a complete obstruction of the artery the blood supply is insufficient to maintain tissue survival. Thus, when the

Figure 7-2   Diagram of the heart and coronary arteries similar to that shown in Figure 7-1 except that now the coronary artery has been completely blocked by further enlargement of the collection of lipid substances in its wall (shown in black). Sometimes such blockage also can happen when a blood clot (thrombosis) forms in a region of the coronary artery that is involved by atherosclerosis ("coronary thrombosis"). When the blood supply to a region of the heart muscle (cross-hatched area) is completely blocked, a portion of that area of muscle will die. The death of the muscle is called a "myocardial infarction"—a result of the coronary occlusion. The cross section of the muscle indicates in black the irregular areas of muscle damage. Often, the outer portion of the wall is spared so that actual rupture of the heart is very infrequent.

Heart Attack
(myocardial infarction, coronary occlusion)

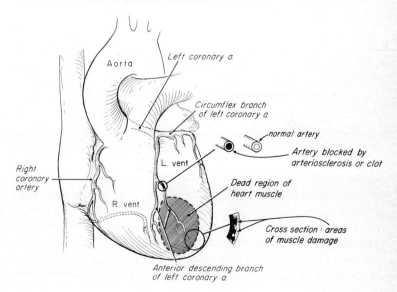

blockage or extreme narrowing occurs, the zone of heart muscle ordinarily supplied with blood by that particular artery, now completely deprived of its oxygen supply, becomes permanently damaged and dies. At that time, very severe chest pain usually is experienced which, in contrast to angina pectoris, often lasts for several hours. Not uncommonly, such an attack occurs in an individual who previously has had few or no symptoms. In other instances, death may come suddenly and without warning, usually as a result of severe electrical disturbance (ventricular fibrillation or cardiac arrest) which may accompany the obstruction of the coronary artery.

It is important to recognize the symptoms of heart attack, since over 40 percent of deaths occur within the first hour after the onset of symptoms, and because about 60 percent of patients who die from a heart attack never reach the hospital. These danger signals are

1 Pressing or squeezing pain, often severe, located behind the lower portion of the breastbone. The pain may radiate or spread to one or both arms, or to the jaw or neck.
2 Sweating often accompanies the pain, and sometimes nausea, vomiting, or shortness of breath occur.

Should such symptoms occur, it is important that an individual reach a doctor or go to a hospital emergency room as soon as possible. It is also important to know that such symptoms often occur in milder form in the hours or days preceding the heart attack itself.

A number of terms are used by physicians to indicate a heart attack, such as "coronary occlusion," "coronary thrombosis" (or simply "a coronary"), and "myocardial infarction." The latter which means death of heart muscle (*myocardium*, meaning heart muscle, *infarction*, meaning death of tissue) is the medical term usually employed.

The effects of blockage of one of the coronary arteries depend in part upon the size of the vessel involved and its location. Occasionally, the zone of muscle supplied by the vessel is so small that no chest pain occurs and the attack goes unrecognized. Sometimes, other blood vessels (termed "collaterals," see below) are able to compensate in part for loss of blood supply by the blocked vessel, the attack may not be noticed by the patient, and an area of old damage may be evident only later, when an electrocardiogram is taken during a routine checkup. As mentioned above, for reasons that are only partially understood, in some cases the damaged area may immediately trigger a severe electrical disturbance of the heart's rhythm which interrupts heart function and is rapidly fatal unless treated within a few minutes. In still other instances, a very large area of muscle may be damaged, a situation that can lead to failure of the pumping action of the heart hours or even days after the patient has reached the hospital. Undoubtedly, one factor of importance in determining the outcome of a heart attack is whether or not other, nearby, blood vessels have a chance to enlarge and to supply tiny new arteries ("collateral" blood vessels) to the involved area (see Figure 3-3). This may have occurred if the coronary artery has been significantly narrowed for a considerable time (perhaps months or years) prior to the attack or, if the patient survives, collaterals develop during the initial hours and days after the complete occlusion. The development of sufficient collateral blood vessels may actually prevent the development of a heart attack, and this factor undoubtedly explains why some patients who have very severe narrowing of several coronary arteries have never experienced a heart attack.

THE TREATMENT OF CORONARY HEART DISEASE

We may consider approaches to the management of this disorder from several aspects, including early identification of high-risk individuals and possible preventive measures, as well as the treatment of patients with chest pain and heart attack. From the long-term study of the population group in Framingham mentioned earlier, a portrait of the "coronary prone" individual and a clearer picture of the importance of various risk factors have gradually emerged. No *single* essential factor has yet been identified, without which the disease fails to occur, but the level of blood pressure, the level of blood lipids (particularly cholesterol), and the blood glucose (diabetic tendency) appear to be three key factors, with age, smoking, and relative body weight also playing important roles. As the degree of abnormality of each of these factors alone or in combination increases, the incidence of coronary heart disease in the population increases. (Of course, if a specific inherited metabolic disease involving the blood lipids exists, the risks are even higher.) Although the tendency for large amounts of saturated fat and cholesterol in the diet to increase blood lipid levels seems established, recent work indicates that the problem is more complicated. Thus, the blood lipid levels in some individuals are now known to be increased by excessive carbohydrates (sugar, starch) in the diet. These individuals may be identified by blood sugar tests, as well as by special patterns of the blood lipids, as discussed below.

Management of the "Coronary Prone" Individual

If the blood pressure is elevated, many effective drugs are now available, and it seems possible that long-term therapy for hypertension will substantially diminish the effects of this risk factor (Chapter 8). Cessation of heavy smoking appears to largely eliminate or reverse the added risk imposed by tobacco. The importance of good general physical condition, while obviously desirable, has not yet been clearly defined, although as mentioned earlier, obesity may provide an added risk. Elevated blood lipids are an important risk factor. When certain fats (lipids) and cholesterol are elevated above normal in the blood, many physicians and scientists now believe that treatment should be instituted in an effort to lower these levels. In addition, many authorities believe that so-called normal blood lipid levels in the United States population are not normal but elevated, at least when compared with lipid levels in populations of certain parts of the world where the incidence of atherosclerosis and coronary heart disease is low. In the United States male population under the age of forty, plasma cholesterol levels exceeding 270 milligrams per 100 milliliters of plasma (mg%) and triglyceride (neutral fat) levels over 150 mg% are considered abnormal. Since the cholesterol level increases with age, sometimes the level of 200 mg% plus the individual's age is taken as a rough guide to the upper limit of normal in younger individuals. Over age 50, cholesterol values exceeding 330 mg% and triglycerides over 190 mg% are considered definitely abnormal, but many physicians and researchers believe that these limits are too high.

Patterns and Treatment of Elevated Cholesterol and Triglycerides in the Blood

Among the abnormalities found in individuals with elevated blood lipids ("hyperlipidemia") several patterns have now been identified. One classification (Fredrickson and Levy) identifies five types, three of which are quite rare and will not be discussed here. Detection and identification of the types in this classification can now be accomplished in most medical laboratories. The basic test consists of observing the movement of certain proteins in the blood plasma to which the lipids are attached ("lipoproteins") when they are placed under the influence of an electrical charge ("electrophoresis"). Recent studies in patients with known coronary heart disease have shown that up to 50 percent may be afflicted with either the Type II or the Type IV pattern (the two most common of the five types). Either of these types appears to occur as an "environmental" form (presumably induced by diet), or as an inherited or familial variety. In Type IV hyperlipidemia, the *triglycerides* are elevated and the cholesterol usually is normal. In Type II the *cholesterol* is elevated and the triglycerides may be normal, but to further complicate matters, subtypes II*a* and II*b* have now been identified; in Type II*a* the cholesterol is high and the triglycerides are normal, but in Type II*b both* the cholesterol and triglycerides are elevated. Type II*a*, so-called familial hypercholesterolemia (high blood cholesterol alone), is inherited as a dominant trait, and one-half of the relatives of an individual with this disorder will carry the gene. Thus, if one parent carries the gene the children have a 50 percent chance of having a high cholesterol level; if *both* parents carry the gene, each child runs a 75 percent risk of having a high cholesterol and a 25 percent risk of being homozygous (having a double dose of the gene). In the latter case, in addition to an elevated blood cholesterol, the child may develop signs of atherosclerosis in childhood and develop premature coronary heart disease in early adult life. When a parent is affected with one of the familial disorders, it therefore becomes important to screen all the children (even infants) for high blood lipid levels, since it is possible that if diet or other treatment is started early enough atherosclerosis may be retarded or even prevented.

Other classifications of abnormal blood lipid patterns have placed emphasis on studying the relatives of patients with coronary heart disease, using only cholesterol and triglyceride measurements, rather than relying on the types determined by electrophoresis discussed above. Thus, it is considered by some investigators that classification using these five types does not distinguish between the environmental and inherited forms of hyperlipidemia. By analyzing lipid levels in patients who had suffered a heart attack as well as their relatives, workers in Seattle, Washington have found that among the 31 percent of the heart attack victims who were found to have hyperlipidemia, more than one-half had a familial or inherited type that was transmitted as a dominant trait. The remaining one-half had either a less clear-cut genetic inheritance pattern, or lipid elevations due to diet and other factors. Thus, about *20 percent of all the heart attack patients proved to have one of the inherited, dominant types of hyperlipidemia.* These familial or inherited forms fell into three groups, associated with either an elevation of cholesterol alone ("familial hypercholesterolemia"—or Type II*a*, discussed above), elevation of triglycerides alone ("familial hypertriglyceridemia"), or with a combined increase in both of these lipids ("familial combined hyperlipidemia"), the latter type being the most common. These investigators emphasize that it is only possible to make this classification if triglyceride and cholesterol levels are measured in a number of the relatives; for example, in the "combined" familial form, the genetic defect may be expressed differently in individuals within the same family—some may have elevation only of the cholesterol, some of the triglycerides, and some of both. Thus, if family studies were not done, or if the electrophoresis typing system only were used, these individuals might be mistakenly classified as familial Types II*a*, Type IV, *or* as one of the nongenetic (environmental) types.

Whatever the best system for categorizing these disorders

proves to be, it is important that the cholesterol *and* triglycerides be examined and the inherited types recognized. Thus, even though the more common inherited forms (familial hypertriglyceridemia and the combined type) usually do not lead to elevated blood lipid levels in childhood, familial hypercholesterolemia does. In the latter condition, the family should be aware that 50 percent of an affected parent's offspring will develop an elevated blood cholesterol, since any approach to management depends on such knowledge. Most of us know at least one family in which premature death from heart attack has involved several generations of fathers, sons, and brothers, and it may be hoped that continued research will produce better understanding and control of these hereditary disorders.

The typical "atherogenic" American diet was discussed in Chapter 4. Special diets have now been developed for the treatment of elevated blood cholesterol and triglycerides, which are *different* for the different patterns of lipid disorders. Two examples can be considered:

In familial *hypercholesterolemia* (Type II hyperlipidemia), often the cholesterol alone is elevated, and it is desirable to reduce particularly the intake of cholesterol and saturated fats. Therefore, total cholesterol intake is markedly reduced to 300 milligrams per day or less (taken only as lean meat), with eggs, organ meats, and shellfish being eliminated from the diet. Pork, beef, and lamb are markedly restricted to reduce intake of saturated (animal) fats, and polyunsaturated fat intake is increased severalfold (using polyunsaturated oils such as safflower, corn, and soy oils, and fish). In such a diet, there is no need to specifically limit carbohydrate intake, alcohol in moderation is permitted, and if the diet does not control the high cholesterol, a drug may be added (see below).

In contrast, in familial *hypertriglyceridemia* (Type IV hyperlipidemia), triglycerides are high and the blood cholesterol is normal. Often there is associated overweight, and there may be a diabetic tendency. In this condition, weight reduction alone sometimes brings the elevated triglycerides down to normal. If not, restriction of carbohydrates in the form of concentrated sugar is necessary, and alcohol (which acts like a carbohydrate and elevates triglyceride levels) should be greatly restricted or eliminated. (In large amounts, alcohol also increases cholesterol levels and can decrease the rate of removal of triglycerides and cholesterol from the bloodstream.) In patients with this disorder, carbohydrates should constitute no more than 40 percent of the total calories, but meat and fat need not be particularly limited, only a moderate increase in polyunsaturated fats is recommended, and cholesterol intake can be more liberal (perhaps 500 mg per day). If these measures are unsuccessful in lowering the triglycerides sufficiently, clofibrate (Atromid-S) often is added to the diet, as discussed below.

In individuals with combined hyperlipidemia (both triglycerides and cholesterol elevated), features of both of the above diets may be used, and Atromid-S may be added. Special cookbooks have become available to assist in the preparation of these various diets in the home (see References).

Several drugs are now available which help to lower the blood lipid levels when diet alone is not sufficient. Cholestyramine and clofibrate are the drugs now used most commonly. Cholestyramine remains in the bowel where it interferes with the absorption of bile salts, thereby increasing their excretion in the stool, apparently at the expense of the body's cholesterol (which shares a common structural unit with these bile acids). Cholesterol in the blood is thereby lowered, even in patients with severe cholesterol elevations of the familial variety. Clofibrate (Atromid-S) interferes with lipid metabolism, lowering primarily the triglycerides and (to a lesser extent) cholesterol. It is useful in individuals with triglyceride elevations of the familial type and in certain patients with combined elevations of cholesterol and triglycerides. Certain other chemicals (so called "chelating agents") have been advocated for use in patients with coronary heart disease in order to remove or "dissolve" the calcium and cholesterol deposits in the arteries. However, there is no good evidence that these agents are of value. In patients with diabetes, often there is associated elevation of the blood lipids. Generally, adequate treatment of the diabetes by diet, insulin, or by other medications which lower the blood sugar levels, results in return of the blood lipids to normal.

In some patients with severe cholesterol elevations of the familial type, a surgical procedure has been performed which involves exclusion of a portion of the intestine where cholesterol absorption is greatest—a portion near the end of the small bowel (ileum). This "ileal bypass" operation can result in considerable weight loss in overweight individuals and also lowers the cholesterol substantially, but its place as a general form of treatment is not yet established.

It will take several years of research to establish firmly whether or not lowering the blood lipids by diet, with our without associated drug treatment, will effectively delay or reverse the atherosclerotic process. Relevant, however, are recent experiments in monkeys which indicate that the accumulation of cholesterol and fatty substances in the walls of blood vessels can be halted or even reversed when previously induced high blood fat lipid levels are reduced by diet or by drugs. Because of such evidence, and that outlined above, most physicians now consider that any individual with elevated blood lipids, whether or not he has coronary heart disease, should be treated with weight reduction (if indicated), a special diet, and one of the aforementioned drugs if necessary. It also seems agreed that other known risk factors such as smoking and high blood pressure should be eliminated or treated.

The Medical Treatment of Chest Pain

For the treatment of patients with angina pectoris, the drug nitroglycerin is available. This agent tends to widen the coronary arteries and improve the heart's blood supply, and even more importantly, it serves to lower the work and oxygen demands on the heart by transient, mild lowering of the blood pressure. Generally, a nitroglycerin tablet placed under the tongue promptly relieves the pain of an attack of angina.

A relatively new type of drug, which often is added when nitroglycerin is insufficient, acts by preventing or blocking the effects of the involuntary nervous system and epinephrine on the heart. By reducing the degree of the increase in heart rate that ordinarily occurs during exercise and by "blocking" the stimulation of the heart muscle caused by nerve impulses to the heart, and by epinephrine from the adrenal glands, the work and oxygen use of the heart are lessened and the frequency and severity of chest pain may be reduced. These drugs, sometimes called "beta-blockers" because of the specific type of chemical receptor in the heart with which they interfere (an example currently available is propranolol, or Inderal), are quite effective in some individuals, or they may be used in combination with nitroglycerin.

The exact place of exercise training in treating patients with angina pectoris, or those who have recovered from a heart attack, has not yet been clearly defined. Whether or not exercise actually results in an improvement of blood flow to the hearts of patients with coronary disease is unknown. However, when it is carefully controlled and increased in a gradual manner, we know that physical conditioning can result in a slower heart rate and more efficient function of the heart, as well as improved efficiency of the muscles of the arms and legs at a given degree of exercise. The work demands on the heart may be reduced thereby, and patients may experience less angina pectoris after such conditioning. It also seems agreed that the unsupervised use of vigorous exercise, particularly in patients with known coronary artery disease, can be hazardous.

Over the years, a number of surgical procedures have been devised in an effort to provide additional blood flow to the hearts of patients with very severe and frequent angina. These so-called revascularization operations have included varied procedures such as implanting the end of an artery (which ordinarily supplies the chest wall) directly into the heart muscle, or the placing of irritating substances (talcum) within the sac around the heart in an effort to cause inflammation and new vascular connections between the heart sac and the heart muscle. The overall success of these two procedures has not been clearly established, although some patients appear to have been benefited. Recently, a highly promising method called "saphenous vein bypass grafting" has been used with increasing frequency throughout the world. In this procedure, a surface vein is taken from the leg (the saphenous vein, the same vein removed in operations for varicose veins), and one end of this vein graft attached to the aorta, the other to the diseased coronary vessel beyond the site of narrowing. Blood is then able to flow from the aorta, through the new channel, and beyond the lipid deposit in the coronary artery (hence the term "bypass graft"), thereby providing oxygenated blood to the heart muscle. The role of this procedure is discussed in Chapter 11. Before the physician considers such an operation, it is necessary to know the location of the narrowed area or areas in the coronary arteries, as well as the condition of the arteries beyond the narrowed area, and therefore x-ray motion pictures with injections of material that can be seen on the x-rays directly into the coronary arteries ("coronary arteriography") is performed prior to considering such procedures. Of course, sometimes such special studies also serve to indicate the *absence* of significant coronary artery disease.

The Treatment of Heart Attack

One of the enormous problems yet to be solved in relation to the treatment of heart attack is the fact that in about 60 percent of the cases, death overtakes the patient at home or en route to a hospital. As mentioned earlier, it is probable that many deaths of this kind result from electrical instability of the heart produced because of the sudden tissue damage, and it is likely that a number of such deaths could be prevented if prompt treatment were available. In some cities, special ambulances having staff trained to give on-the-scene treatment of heart attack and containing equipment for applying electrical shocks to "defibrillate" the heart (Chapter 6) are undergoing trials to determine their practicability. If the patient reaches the hospital, the likelihood of his surviving the acute heart attack are reasonably good (about eight chances in ten), although this figure depends on factors such as age, the size of the zone of heart muscle involved, and how many previous heart attacks have occurred.

The treatment of heart attack has undergone important advances in the past few years, most important being the establishment of monitoring of the electrocardiogram by specially trained nursing staff in the coronary care unit ("CCU"). By continuously observing the electrocardiogram for two to four days after the attack, many serious electrical disturbances of the heart's rhythm can be prevented by medication, and those that do occur often can be treated effectively. The occurrence of frequent extra heartbeats, a sign which may precede more serious electrical disorders, can be detected and abolished promptly with appropriate medications, before a serious complication develops. Heart block, which may result from damage to the heart's conduction system, can be rapidly detected in its earliest forms and when necessary treated by an electrical pacemaker. Two catastrophic events that formerly caused sudden death, even in the hospital, before the advent of the CCU are cardiac arrest and "ventricular fibrillation." Arrest, or absence of electrical activity, often progresses to ventricular fibrillation which is a very rapid, completely disordered, and ineffective motion of the muscle of the pumping chambers. Both of these potentially fatal rhythm disturbances can be treated promptly by an electrical shock applied across the chest, a procedure which can be performed in the modern coronary care unit within one minute after such a disorder is detected. The staff in such a unit also can maintain the circulation by regular external compressions of the chest ("external cardiac massage") and by artificial respiration if such electrical shocks are not immediately effective.

If the area of muscle damage is especially large, the heart may fail in its pumping function in the early hours or days after a heart attack, and the patient may develop a low blood pressure, or shock. Considerable research is now underway on new drugs to support the circulation and strengthen the heart under these circumstances, as well as on possible ways to reduce the ultimate size of the damaged area. Artificial support devices to tide the patient over the period of heart failure and shock are sometimes employed (Chapter 11). One example of such an artificial support system currently used in some centers for patients with heart attack complicated by shock is called "balloon counterpulsation." A small flexible tube (catheter) is inserted through an artery in the leg and positioned within the aorta inside the chest. A balloon at the end of the tube is electronically triggered from the electrocardiogram to inflate and deflate in time with the heart's cycle, so that during the rest phase of the cycle the balloon inflates inside the aorta, forcing blood backward against the closed aortic valve and thereby helping to push blood through the coronary arteries to nourish the heart muscle. However, during the contracting phase of the heart cycle, the balloon rapidly deflates to lower the blood pressure and thereby reduce the work demands on the pumping chamber. This device has been effective for temporary support f the circulation for hours, or even days, in patients whose heart attack is so severe that the blood pressure cannot be maintained. While receiving such temporary support, a few patients have now been saved from almost certain death by carrying out an emergency operation, a vein graft bypass procedure to the blocked coronary arteries. Such measures are currently carried out in only a few medical centers and are reserved for patients who have suffered a massive heart attack and show little hope of recovery.

In most patients, healing occurs after a heart attack. Generally, a period of rest of two or three weeks is advised to allow time for the formation of scar tissue in the area of damaged muscle. The scar formation is well along at the end of this time and is usually complete after five or six weeks. A period of gradual increase in activity usually is then recommended, the patient being able to return to his normal activities in about two months. This recovery sequence is the rule in most patients following their first heart attack, although the time periods may be shorter if the area of damage has been small, and longer if the attack was a severe one. In some patients, particularly those who have suffered several previous heart attacks, or a large area of damage, difficulties with angina pectoris or heart failure may persist after a heart attack. Under these circumstances, surgical treatment is sometimes then advised.

REFERENCES

General

Ames, R., "How to Survive a Heart Attack," *Reader's Digest*, November 1973.

American Heart Association Cookbook, David McKay, New York, 1973.

Blakeslee, A., and Stamler, J., *Your Heart Has Nine Lives*, Prentice-Hall, Inc., Englewood Cliffs, N.J., 1966.

Blumenfeld, A., *Heart Attack. Are You a Candidate?*, Paul S. Eriksson, Inc., New York, 1964.

Clark, M., "Curbing the Killer," *Newsweek*, May 1, 1972.

1973 Heart Facts (E. M. 509*A*), American Heart Association, New York, 1973 (pamphlet).

Reduce Your Risk of Heart Attack (E. M. 392), American Heart Association, New York, 1969 (pamphlet).

Rescue Breathing to Save a Life (E. M. 446), American Heart Association, New York 1971 (pamphlet).

Scientific Works

Fredrickson, D. S., "A Physician's Guide to Hyperlipidemia," *Modern Concepts of Cardiovascular Disease*, **41**:31, 1972.

Friedberg, C. K., *Acute Myocardial Infarction and Coronary Care Units*, Grune & Stratton, New York, 1969.

Friedman, M., *Pathogenesis of Coronary Artery Disease*, McGraw-Hill, New York, 1969.

Fox, S. M., Naughton, J. P., and Gorman, P. A., "Physical Activity in Cardiovascular Health," *Modern Concepts in Cardiovascular Disease*, **41**:13, 1972.

Goldstein, J. L., Hazzard, W. R., Schrott, H. G., Bierman, E. L., and Motulsky, A. G., "Genetics of Hyperlipidemia in Coronary Heart Disease," *Transactions of the Association of American Physicians*, **85**:120, 1972.

Lesch, M., and Gorlin, R., "Pharmacological Therapy of Angina Pectoris," *Modern Concepts of Cardiovascular Disease*, **42**:5, 1973.

Pitt, D. and Ross, R. S., "Beta-Adrenergic Blockade in Cardiovascular Therapy," *Modern Concepts of Cardiovascular Disease*, **38**:47, 1969.

Shapter, R. K., "Cardiopulmonary Resuscitation: Basic Life Support," *Clinical Symposia*, **26**:4–31, 1974.

White, P. D., and Donovan, H., *Hearts. Their Long Follow-up*, W. B. Saunders, Philadelphia, 1967.

High Blood Pressure

Direct blood pressure measurements date back to 1733 when the Englishman Stephen Hales determined the blood pressure in living horses by placing a small tube into an artery and connecting it to a pipe. He then measured the vertical height of the column of blood within the tube (about seventy inches). The indirect cuff method used today in the physician's office to measure the systolic and diastolic pressures is described in Chapter 1 (see Figure 1-2). High blood pressure (hypertension) is recognized as an abnormally elevated blood pressure, frequently associated with structural and functional abnormalities of many organs, particularly the blood vessels, the heart, the brain, and kidneys.

The Normal Blood Pressure

Any change in the output of blood by the heart would be associated with a change in blood pressure in the same direction unless an opposing change occurred in the resistance to blood flow by either relaxation or contraction of the small resistance arteries. To use an analogy employed previously, when a garden hose is constricted, pressure rises in the hose on the side nearest the faucet when the faucet is opened more widely. In healthy subjects, the blood pressure remains within a relatively narrow range (about 30 percent above or below its normal resting value) despite large alterations in heart output (from one-third below to five times above its resting level). Clearly, then, regulation of the blood pressure by the resistance blood vessels normally is present. During the course of daily activities, many factors can influence the blood pressure: body posture, exercise, gastrointestinal activity, emotion or painful stimuli, environmental factors (temperature, noise level), and coffee, tobacco, or drugs; all can have direct or indirect effects on the caliber of the small arteries or the output of blood by the heart. However, the effects of these sudden influences are buffered in the normal individual by reflexes which operate through the involuntary nervous system and regulate the caliber of these blood vessels.

The normal blood pressure range is a set of pressure limits derived statistically from pressure values in a randomly selected segment of the population. This normal range is sometimes defined as two standard deviations on either side of the population mean (which includes 95 percent of the population). Since blood pressure levels vary with age, sex, or racial groupings, the normal range differs in various population groups. Most commonly, the blood pressure limits are chosen by defining arbitrarily a given percentage of subjects above and below the mean as normal, borderline, or elevated.

The blood pressure increases rapidly over the first few days of life and then rises gradually throughout life, the increment in systolic pressure (the maximum pressure in each beat) being slightly greater than the diastolic pressure (the lowest pressure in each beat). The average blood pressure tends to be higher in Western industrialized societies than in underdeveloped countries. The normal upper limits of blood pressure for adults in our society are approximately 140 millimeters of mercury for systolic pressure and 90 millimeters of mercury for diastolic pressure. In an individual subject, however, baseline pressure values above these normal limits do not necessarily indicate an abnormal state of hypertension, since the physiologic range of normal for an individual occasionally extends into the statistical range of abnormal for the total population. Somewhat higher systolic blood pressures than 140 millimeters of mercury (up to 160 or even 170) are accepted as normal in older individuals.

Causes of High Blood Pressure

In most subjects, the finding of a *diastolic* blood pressure consistently above 90 millimeters of mercury usually represents hypertension. High blood pressure can arise from several different disorders which either increase blood flow, the resistance to blood flow, or both. Elevation of the systolic and diastolic blood pressure consistently, over long periods of time, however, is almost always due primarily to an abnormally high resistance to blood flow in the small arteries of the systemic circulation (Figure 8-1). Sometimes the blood pressure is only intermittently elevated; it is unsettled as to whether or not such *labile hypertension* usually leads to the permanent variety, although this appears to be the case in some individuals.

It is estimated that 10 to 15 percent of the general population has an abnormally elevated blood pressure. In 85 percent of these patients, no specific cause for the high blood pressure can be found, and a diagnosis of *essential hypertension* is made. In the remaining 15 percent of patients with an elevated blood pressure a specific disease process is identified, and the diagnosis of *secondary hypertension* is established. The causes of secondary hypertension in this smaller group of patients include such problems as kidney disease, which can result from long-standing infection, diabetes, disease of the blood vessels supplying the kidney, or other processes leading to kidney damage; tumors of the pituitary or adrenal glands which release excessive amounts of hormones that can cause hypertension (these tumors often can be removed surgically); or an inborn constriction of the aorta (coarctation), which also is amenable to surgical correction (see Chapter 10). A careful search for such secondary causes of hypertension usually is made.

In the great majority of patients with hypertension, however,

High Blood Pressure

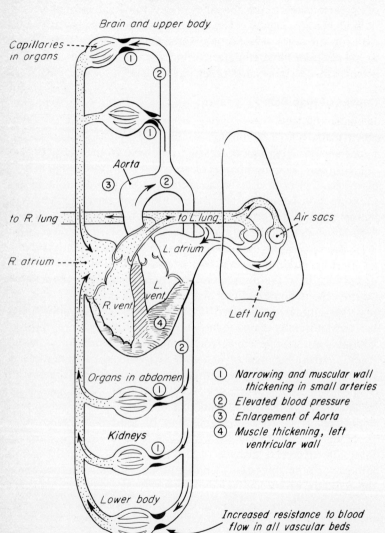

① Narrowing and muscular wall
   thickening in small arteries
② Elevated blood pressure
③ Enlargement of Aorta
④ Muscle thickening, left
   ventricular wall

Increased resistance to blood
flow in all vascular beds
caused by narrowing

no specific cause is identified, although there is increasing evidence that such *essential hypertension* tends to run in families and is very likely a genetic disorder. Physicians who have observed families with a high incidence of stroke associated with elevated blood pressure have long been aware of this familial clustering of essential hypertension. Scientific studies of patterns of inheritance of this disorder also support the conclusion that essential hypertension is genetically transmitted. Racial differences in the incidence of hypertension also have been investigated, and there is little doubt that in biracial communities of the United States hypertension is more frequent in the black population. It also appears that the disease is more severe among blacks.

Hormones and High Blood Pressure

As mentioned earlier, it is established that when diastolic blood pressure consistently is elevated there is an excessive resistance to flow of blood through the small arteries. Although numerous factors can affect the caliber of the small arteries, of primary importance is the substance norepinephrine, which is contained within special nerve fibers located in the walls of the small arteries. This hormone is also found in the adrenal gland. The reflexes of the involuntary (autonomic) nervous system normally regulate the amount of norepinephrine release in the blood vessel walls on a moment to moment basis. When increased amounts of this hormone are released by the nerves, a marked reduction in the caliber of the small arteries (arterial constriction) occurs which leads to increased resistance to flow, and hence elevates the blood pressure.

Another hormone, aldosterone, which is secreted normally

Figure 8-1 Changes which occur in the circulation in the presence of hypertension or high blood pressure (compare with Figure 1-1). The narrowed areas (labeled 1) in the blood vessels supplying the various organs constitute the primary abnormality; that is, there is an increased resistance to blood flow in all the small arteries of the body. This causes elevation of the blood pressure in the aorta and other large arteries of the body (labeled 2). Complications of longstanding high blood pressure consist of thickening of the wall of the left ventricle, or left-sided pumping chamber (labeled 4), and sometimes an aneurysm or enlargement of the aorta (labeled 3).

by the adrenal glands also plays a significant role in the control of blood pressure. Oversecretion of this hormone is accompanied by a retention of the sodium ion by the body, an increase in the volume of blood contained within the circulation, and an elevation of the blood pressure. The mechanism of the effect of this hormone on the blood pressure is not completely understood, but an overload of ingested sodium may cause hypertension in some patients, particularly those who have impaired circulatory regulation (heart failure).

A third hormone of major importance in the regulation of blood pressure is the substance renin, a protein material normally released from the kidney, which reacts with a precursor contained in the blood to produce still another substance called "angiotensin." Angiotensin increases the blood pressure by causing constriction of the small arteries, and in addition it stimulates aldosterone secretion by the adrenal gland, leading to sodium retention as well. Normally, the levels of all these hormones are closely regulated by the nervous system and the body's complex hormonal regulatory mechanisms to maintain an appropriate level of blood pressure for the level of activity or physiologic state.

When these body systems fail, excessive secretion of norepinephrine, aldosterone, or renin can result in persistent elevation of the blood pressure. For example, in patients with hypertension secondary to certain types of tumors of the adrenal gland, the elevated blood pressure results from increased norepinephrine secretion by the tumor (pheochromocytoma), or with other types of adrenal tumor, from excessive aldosterone secretion. In patients with high blood pressure secondary to kidney diesase, or from narrowing of a blood vessel supplying the kidney, the elevated blood pressure results from increased release of renin and activation of the angiotensin-aldosterone system. In the large number of patients who have *essential hypertension*, however, the specific reason for the inadequate regulation of the blood pressure is still unknown. Despite this uncertainty as to precise cause, certain modern drugs which interfere with or block the operation of one or more of these nervous and endocrine regulatory systems have been used with outstanding success in the treatment of essential hypertension, as discussed further below.

How Is High Blood Pressure Detected?

Essential hypertension usually becomes manifest between the ages of thirty and forty years, although it is by no means rare for the disease to begin earlier. The clinical diagnosis is made by the indirect measurement of the systolic and diastolic arterial pressures with a pneumatic cuff (Figure 1-2). Frequently, the elevated diastolic blood pressure is detected during a routine physical examination in a patient who has absolutely no symptoms. For this reason, and because of the serious complications of untreated long-standing high blood pressure, "hypertension detection clinics" have been established by the American Heart Association and its local affiliates. A smaller number of patients with hypertension consult a physician because of symptoms due to the effects of the high blood pressure itself. These symptoms include recurrent morning headaches, frequent nose bleeds, and difficulties such as weakness, nervousness, heart palpitations or dizziness. More severe symptoms occur, of course, as the patient develops heart or brain complications from long-standing, untreated hypertension.

Complications of High Blood Pressure

With persistent diastolic pressure elevation, regardless of its cause, the small arteries of the body constitute the initial focus for its damaging effect. In early hypertension the small arteries appear normal under the microscope, but later there is abnormal thickening of the muscular wall of the smallest arteries. This change is followed by a progressive decrease in the size of the channel within these vessels. In general, there is a relationship between the extent of such pathologic changes in the arteries and the severity of the blood pressure elevation, and with very marked hypertension, localized areas of complete destruction involving all layers of the arterial wall eventually occur. These changes may occur in any and all parts of the circulation, including the coronary arteries supplying the heart, the vessels of the eye (retina), and those to the kidney and brain. Small areas of cell and tissue death may occur in these organs as a result of inadequate blood supply, the result of narrowing and damage to the blood vessels (Figure 8-1). In addition, a consistently elevated blood pressure may affect larger arteries through its tendency to stimulate atherosclerosis, the formation of yellowish plaques containing cholesterol and fats on the inner wall of the arteries. By accelerating this process, persistent hypertension may further adversely affect the blood supply to the heart, the kidneys, and the brain.

High blood pressure also affects the heart muscle, causing thickening (hypertrophy) of the left ventricular wall. This results from increased muscle protein synthesis, stimulated by the increased workload placed on this pumping chamber by the high systolic blood pressure required during each heartbeat. In addition, as mentioned, coronary artery disease and complications of angina pectoris and heart attack are observed with increased frequency in hypertensive patients. Another complication of hypertension which commonly occurs is heart failure, attended by enlargement of the left ventricle and congestion in the lungs, the result of damage to the heart muscle from long-standing overwork (Figure 8-1).

In hypertensive subjects, the aorta becomes enlarged, and thickening or destruction of the muscle in its wall often occurs. Sometimes, rupture of an area of outpouching of the aortic wall (aneurysm, see Figure 8-1) occurs, resulting in bleeding into the chest, or even sudden death. The complications in the kidney due to high blood pressure are primarily related to the abnormalities in the small arteries described previously. As a consequence of an inadequate blood supply, the kidneys may have poor function, and actual destruction of localized areas of kidney tissue often results.

The complications of hypertension which affect the brain are numerous. The earliest changes can be seen only with the microscope and consist of destruction of small areas of brain tissue due to poor blood supply. There is a marked increase in the incidence of stroke in patients with high blood pressure, and a large zone of brain tissue may be damaged by such an occurrence. Strokes are due to severe damage and narrowing of the small arteries supplying the brain which leads to an insufficient cerebral blood flow, to bleeding into the brain substance due to a ruptured blood vessel, or to atherosclerosis and blockage of one of the larger blood vessels which supply the brain.

Treatment of High Blood Pressure

If one of the secondary causes for hypertension can be found, surgical removal of an adrenal tumor or a coarctation at the aorta usually cures the problem. Sometimes, if an artery to the kidney is narrowed, hypertension can be cured by surgically relieving the narrowing. If other types of kidney disease involve only one of the kidneys, hypertension occasionally is cured by removing that kidney. Sometimes, however, if the high blood pressure has been long-standing, relieving a narrowed artery to the kidney, or other surgical treatment, may be ineffective because of damage by the hypertension to the small blood vessels of both kidneys.

The aim of effective drug therapy for hypertension is to control both systolic and diastolic blood pressure at strictly normal levels, twenty-four hours a day, and to prevent the onset and progression of blood vessel damage. Medical treatment, including a low-salt diet and the administration of various pharmacologic agents, can be highly effective in the control of high blood pressure. Drugs used in the treatment of hypertension include diuretic agents which increase the excretion of sodium by the kidneys; drugs such as reserpine and methyldopa which decrease the effect of norepinephrine on the small arteries, thereby increasing their caliber; agents such as hydralazine which produce dilatation of the small arteries; drugs which block the effect of the hormone aldosterone on the kidney thereby decreasing salt retention; and the beta-adrenergic blocking agent propranolol which reduces the output of blood by the heart. Each of these deserves brief mention.

Thiazide diuretics commonly are used as the sole therapy in patients with mild hypertension, or they may be used in conjunction with other antihypertensive drugs in patients whose blood pressure is not controlled by diuretics alone. The mechanism by which these agents lower blood pressure is not clearly understood. It may be related to a decrease in the volume of blood in the circulation, to loss of sodium by the kidneys, or to a direct dilating effect on the small arteries. The reduction of blood pressure may not occur unless there is increased urine volume resulting from the use of these agents. The effective dose depends upon kidney function, and to some extent on the salt intake.

Reserpine, a drug obtained from the root of the *Rauwolfia serpentina* plant, is widely used in the treatment of mild or moderate blood pressure elevation. Its primary effect is to impair the storage of norepinephrine within the sympathetic nerve terminals, thereby decreasing the narrowing of the small arteries which results from norepinephrine release by the nerves.

Methyldopa (Aldomet) is a frequently used drug, the antihypertensive effect of which may be related to displacement of norepinephrine from the sympathetic nerve terminals. Methyldopa is most useful in patients whose blood pressure is not satisfactorily controlled by the thiazides, or by the combination of thiazide and reserpine.

Hydralazine (Apresoline) reduces the arterial blood pressure by decreasing the resistance to blood flow in the small arteries (dilating them). Hydralazine sometimes is added when the blood pressure does not respond to thiazide-reserpine or thiazide-methyldopa therapy. Because of its propensity to cause an increase in the heart's output of blood and heart rate, it usually is not used in patients with severe coronary heart disease or heart failure, since an increase in the workload of the heart may aggravate their heart symptoms.

Guanethidine (Ismelin) is a potent drug which is used for the treatment of patients with moderately severe or severe hypertension. It acts by preventing the release of norepinephrine from the sympathetic nerve terminals, thereby increasing the caliber of the small arteries. Because guanethidine is a potent drug and often causes a severe drop in systolic blood pressure when the patient stands up, this agent must be given with great care.

Spironolactone (Aldactone) is an inhibitor of aldosterone, the hormone released from the adrenal gland which results in salt and water retention. Spironolactone is sometimes a useful adjunct in the treatment of patients with essential hypertension.

Propranolol hydrochloride (Inderal) is a beta-adrenergic blocking agent which exerts a mild to moderate hypotensive effect, probably due to a reduction in systemic blood flow (cardiac output). At present it appears to be useful particularly in patients with high blood pressure accompanied by chest pain due to coincident coronary artery disease. The combination of propranolol, hydralazine, and a diuretic often is effective in patients with moderate to severe hypertension who cannot tolerate or have failed to respond to other drugs, the propranolol serving to block the heart rate–increasing effect of the hydralazine.

Does Lowering Blood Pressure Reduce Risk?

A cooperative study concerning the effects of adequate high blood pressure treatment on the complications of hypertension has recently been completed at the Veterans Administration hospitals. A total of 380 hypertensive male patients with diastolic blood pressures of 90 to 114 millimeters of mercury were randomly assigned to either a no-treatment group or to an active antihypertensive-therapy program. The risk of developing a serious complication from hypertension was reduced by treatment from 55 percent to 18 percent over a five-year period. Nineteen deaths due to hypertension or atherosclerosis ("hardening of the arteries") occurred in the untreated group, but there were only eight deaths in the actively treated group. In addition, twenty untreated patients developed very high diastolic blood pressures of 125 millimeters of mercury or more. Treatment was more effective in preventing congestive heart failure and stroke than in preventing the complications of coronary artery disease in this relatively short-term study, but it seems possible that with adequate treatment of hypertension over many years, the accelerated rate or progression of atherosclerosis associated with high blood pressure will be markedly slowed or even stopped.

It can be concluded that effective treatment is unquestionably beneficial in preventing complications and death related to the abnormally elevated blood pressure.

REFERENCES

General

Cerebral Vascular Disease and Strokes, U.S. Department of Health, Education and Welfare. Public Health Service, National Institutes of Health, 1969.

Hypertension, High Blood Pressure, Heart Information Center, National Heart Institute, Bethesda, Md., 1969.

Hypertension—High Blood Pressure (No. 1714), Heart Information Center, National Heart Institute, National Institutes of Health, 1969.

1973 Heart Facts (E. M. 509A), American Heart Association, New York, 1973 (pamphlet).

Stamler, J., Stamler, R., and Pullman, T. N., *The Epidemiology of Hypertension*, Grune & Stratton, New York, 1967.

Scientific Works

Freis, E. D., "Medical Treatment of Chronic Hypertension," *Modern Concepts in Cardiovascular Disease*, **40**:17, 1971.

"Veterans Administration Cooperative Study Group on Antihypertensive Agents: Effects of Treatment on Morbidity and Hypertension: Results in Patients with Diastolic Blood Pressure Averaging 115 through 129 mmHg," *Journal of the American Medical Association*, **202**:1028, 1967.

"Veterans Administration Cooperative Study Group on Antihypertensive Agents: Effects of Treatment and Morbidity in Hypertension II: Results in Patients with Diastolic Blood Pressure Averaging 90 through 115 mmHg," *Journal of the American Medical Association*, **213**:1143, 1970.

Chapter 9

Heart Failure and Diseases of Heart Muscle

In this chapter we will discuss how abnormalities of the subsystems of the heart described in previous chapters (the electrical conduction system, the coronary arteries, the heart valves) and other diseases can lead to damage of the muscle of the heart. Often this damage results from long-standing overwork of the heart muscle or from actual loss of muscle tissue (as with a heart attack). Eventually, the overworked heart then fails in its function as a pump. In addition, certain disease processes can directly affect the muscle cells of the heart causing them to fail in their contractile function.

The Causes of Heart Failure

Primary Diseases of the Heart Muscle Just as there are diseases which specifically affect nervous tissue (such as the virus of poliomyelitis), so certain diseases can directly affect the muscle of the heart (*myocardial disease*, from the Greek terms for muscle, and *kardia*, or heart). Such diseases of heart muscle can be due to viral or other infections, but most are of uncertain cause, or secondary to an illness elsewhere in the body. When viruses or bacteria invade the heart muscle, the process is called a "myocarditis," and when they invade the sac that surrounds the heart, the infection that results is called "pericarditis." Such infectious agents may kill the muscle cells, leading to loss of muscle tissue and scar formation with permanent heart damage, but more often (as with other tissues affected by viruses or bacteria) healing of the tissue and complete recovery occur. Nevertheless, it is possible that some patients who later develop heart failure due to disease of the heart muscle of uncertain cause may in fact be in a late stage of a previously unrecognized viral infection, no longer active, but which caused severe damage. Others may have suffered an unrecognized toxic or allergic reaction involving the heart. For example, it is known that the inflammation of the heart muscle which accompanies acute rheumatic fever is an allergic response to the streptococcus. Severe alcoholism has been shown to result in damage to the muscle fibers and eventually to impairment of heart function. Rare diseases of an allergic type that affect very small blood vessels supplying the heart also can cause severe damage to the heart muscle. However, the cause of the majority of cases of "primary" heart muscle disease (involving *only* the muscle cells of the heart) remains unknown.

Other Causes of Heart Failure   The most common conditions which ultimately lead to weakness and failure of the heart muscle, as a secondary phenomenon, may be listed with reference to the heart's subsystems:

1 *Electrical failure of the heart.* When the electrical conduction system of the heart is damaged and heart block occurs, lack of conduction between the pacemaker of the heart (located in the receiving chambers) and the ventricles results in a very slow ventricular beating rate, which eventually can lead to a low output of blood from the heart and to heart failure. When the heart rate is extremely low (about forty-five beats per minute) the heart enlarges in compensation, and thereby delivers a larger amount of blood for each beat. Eventually this increased burden can result in damage to the muscle; in addition, often there is associated disease of the coronary arteries in these patients, many of whom are elderly. Implantation of a permanent electrical cardiac pacemaker, together with other treatment for the failing heart muscle described below, usually serves to correct this form of heart failure.

   2   When there is disease of the *coronary arteries*, numerous small areas of damage occurring over the years, or a single large heart attack, may result in replacement of the heart muscle to a large extent by scar tissue. Failure of the left-sided pumping chamber then ensues.

   3   *Valvular heart disease*, particularly of the left-sided valves (the aortic and mitral valve) with narrowing or leakage of either or both valves, results in enlargement of the heart in order to compensate for the necessary extra work. Eventually, after a number of years, small areas of scar tissue tend to form in the heart muscle and, again, failure of the heart may ensue.

   4   *High blood pressure*, another condition which causes overwork of the left-sided pumping chamber, leads to enlargement of the wall of that chamber. Eventually, if the high blood pressure persists over many years, the heart muscle weakens and failure occurs.

Thus, the end result of these diverse diseases is poor function of the heart due to weakness of its muscular wall. Early during the course of these disease processes, the body and heart are able to compensate for weakness of the heart muscle. These initial compensations occur in two primary ways:

   1   The heart becomes larger. Initially its enlargement brings about increased stretch on the muscle fibers, which allows them to develop more force and to deliver a larger amount of blood (see Starling's law, increased stretch on the muscle causing increased interaction of the protein filaments within the muscle, Chapter 2). Also, over the months and years *more* muscle tissue is produced (sometimes called "hypertrophy"). This process produces new muscle by protein synthesis to replace scarred muscle, or to bolster weakened muscle, and such enlargement of the heart may become quite extreme. This chronic enlargement, although eventually detrimental, may for a time allow the weakened heart to maintain its output of blood with each beat. The simple analogy relative to the benefits of such heart enlargement is to consider a rubber balloon. If the balloon is enlarged and distended with water, a very slight squeeze of the balloon with the fingers will deliver an amount of fluid out of the neck of the balloon that would require a much larger degree of compression if the balloon were much smaller and only half filled. In a similar manner, the greatly enlarged heart can deliver an amount of blood per beat that may be nearly normal, despite weakened and reduced contraction of its muscular wall.

2   The nervous system comes into play. When the heart begins to fail, nerve receptors in the blood vessels, the heart, and in the brain sense the inadequate output of blood from the heart and activate the sympathetic nervous system (part of the "involuntary" nervous system). This system then delivers electrical impulses along the nerve network directed to the heart causing release of the substance norepinephrine contained within the nerve endings, which lie among the heart muscle fibers. As described in Chapter 2, this substance, together with epinephrine released into the circulation from the adrenal glands which lie near the kidneys, stimulates the heart muscle. Both the rate of beating of the heart and the strength of contraction of the heart muscle are thereby increased. Ultimately, however, this and other compensatory mechanisms break down, and despite maximum treatment with medication, swelling in the lungs and tissues begins and the patient may die from heart failure.

What Are the Effects of Heart Failure?   Since the heart is really two pumps, the right-sided pump, the left-sided pump, or both may fail. When the left side of the heart fails for any of a variety of reasons, it becomes unable to pump enough blood forward. The patient may at first feel muscle fatigue on exertion, the heart being unable to deliver sufficient blood flow to the exercising muscles to meet their demands for oxygen. In addition, just as when a water pump becomes faulty, increased pressure builds up behind the failing pump. In the case of the left heart, such elevated pressure is transmitted backward into the lungs through the blood vessels leading to the heart, raising the pressure inside the smallest blood vessels in the lungs, the capillaries (see Figure 1-1). These tiny vessels are so thin-walled that fluid from the blood filters out into the tissues of the lungs and accumulates between the air sacs. This leads to increased stiffness of the lungs, increases the work of breathing, and the patient complains of shortness of breath. Shortness of breath often becomes worse when patients lie down or when they perform exercise, since both of these situations cause a further increase in the back pressure. When the pressure in the capillaries becomes very high, fluid may leak directly into the air sacs, producing coughing and breathing difficulty. In severe cases, the back pressure may be transmitted through the lungs and cause overloading on the right-sided pumping chamber.

In individuals with severe lung disorders such as emphysema, the right heart alone may fail late in the course of the disease. In this situation, as in certain types of inborn heart disease, the pressure in the arteries *leading to* the lungs (pulmonary arteries) becomes elevated, resulting in overwork of the right ventricle (Figure 1-1). As with left-sided failure, a buildup of pressure behind the failing right ventricle then occurs which is, in this case transmitted backward into the veins of the body. If severe enough, the elevated pressure leads to leakage of fluid which accumulates particularly in the ankles and lower legs. As in left-sided failure, this fluid is a filtrate of blood containing no blood cells, and having a low protein content. In extreme right heart failure, leakage of fluid may occur into the abdomen causing it to swell, and the swelling of the legs (termed "edema") may extend all the way up to the waist. In olden times such generalized swelling was called "dropsy," now recognized to have several causes in addition to heart failure (kidney disease, liver disease).

Why Do Heart Muscle Cells Become Weak?   As shown in Figure 2-5, the protein strands in heart muscle slide past one another and active sites on the protein filaments interact to allow force to be generated and the heart to eject blood. One early theory of the cause of heart failure was that as the heart enlarged an overstretching and perhaps even an actual disengagement of the filaments in heart muscle could occur and thereby prevent contact between the active chemical sites. Recently, however, studies in experimental heart failure using the electron microscope have shown that even with very severe enlargement of the heart this is not the case. The filaments do not appear to be pulled apart, and therefore this explanation of the weakness of the muscle is incorrect.

Some of the most promising clues to the basic problem in failing heart muscle have been provided by studies of certain important ions (such as calcium) which move within the heart muscle during each heart cycle. Within the cell there is a large store of calcium contained in a network of tiny tubules which surround the protein filaments, as well as calcium that is bound to sites on the inside of the cell wall. In some way, each electrical impulse when it arrives at the cell causes release of this calcium, and the free calcium moves in among the thick and thin protein filaments in the muscle, causing them to contract. It appears that one calcium ion activates each chemical binding site on the protein filaments, so that when more calcium reaches the contractile protein filaments, more bonds are activated and the muscle can beat more strongly. Conversely, a reduction in the release of calcium causes a weaker contraction. This sequence of events probably is of great importance in understanding, at the molecular level, how heart muscle fails, since experiments have shown that there may be faulty calcium release and uptake in damaged heart muscle.

The precise means by which calcium initiates the contraction of muscle is not entirely clear. One possibility is that when the calcium reaches the chemical site, it binds directly to a special protein in the filament, a protein that ordinarily "covers" the active site when the heart is in the rest phase of its cycle. The binding of the calcium could cause a change in the shape of the special protein, which uncovers the chemical site. The active site can then interact with the opposite filament, and the muscle contracts and shortens. This central role of calcium in heart muscle contraction is discussed further below with reference to an important drug that is used to treat heart failure: digitalis.

The Treatment of Heart Failure

When heart failure is caused by damage to one of the heart's subsystems, it sometimes can be reversed by special forms of treatment such as insertion of an artificial heart valve, placement of an electrical pacemaker, or bypass grafting for a diseased coronary artery as described in other chapters. Usually heart failure can be relieved in the patient with high blood pressure by treating the hypertension with appropriate drugs, thereby relieving the work overload on the heart. If such definitive forms of treatment are not feasible, as is the case when heart failure is due to extensive and permanent damage of the heart muscle, supportive treatment with various medications is undertaken. Undoubtedly, some patients with end-stage heart failure eventually will become candidates for surgical replacement of the heart, if this procedure ever becomes widely applicable (Chapter 11). Short of this, treatment with drugs such as diuretics and digitalis greatly benefits many patients.

Because of poor blood supply to the kidneys and certain hormonal imbalances that occur in heart failure, the kidneys tend to excrete salt poorly. This, in turn, causes the body to retain water and further aggravates the tendency for fluid to build up in the tissues of the legs and the lungs of patients with heart failure. Therefore, the patient must reduce his salt (sodium chloride) intake. In addition, there are now many potent "diuretics" which promote the excretion of fluid via the kidneys. These drugs affect the kidney tissue directly to cause loss of sodium ion into the urine, and this ion carries water with it thereby removing excess fluid from the tissues. Potassium ion also is lost, and often this must be replaced by taking foods or medications which have a high content of potassium. When used regularly, diuretics are highly effective in the treatment of heart failure.

The Story of Digitalis   This important drug was known to the Egyptians as an extract of a plant called the sea onion (the drug was termed "squill"), and even in Roman times it was known to be a heart tonic and to cause increased passage of urine. Because of its toxic effects on the heart when ingested in very large doses, it also was used as a rat poison. In Africa, digitalis in another form (also a plant extract) was used to poison arrow tips; very high doses were an effective weapon, since poisoning by digitalis can cause the heart to stop beating.

The first formal Western writings about digitalis were in 1785 by William Withering, an English physician. He had heard of the effectiveness of the drug for the treatment of "dropsy" (generalized swelling of the body) from an old woman who was using the powdered leaves of a common garden plant, the foxglove. The active agent in this plant was called *Digitalis purpurea* (because of the finger-like shape of the purple flower), and Withering found it to be a very effective treatment indeed for many cases of dropsy. Unlike the Romans, however, he did not realize that the major reason for its effectiveness in these cases was its tonic effect on the heart, although he did notice that it increased the force of the heartbeat. It seems likely that those cases of dropsy that he reported which did *not* respond to digitalis under his treatment were due to kidney or liver disease.

Digitalis continues to be used widely because of its effect, in low doses, to markedly strengthen the beat of the failing heart. Although other medications such as epinephrine and norepinephrine (discussed earlier), which occur naturally in the body, are potent stimulators of the failing heart, they are broken down very rapidly in the body. Moreover, they cannot be taken by mouth because of their rapid destruction in the gastrointestinal tract. Digitalis is effective when taken in pill form, and it has a very long duration of action (one dose lasting several days), properties which have led to its wide application in treating patients with heart failure. Digitalis commonly is prescribed in several forms. It is still available as the powdered digitalis leaf, but more commonly synthetic types called "digitoxin" and "digoxin" are used. This drug also is effective for slowing excessively rapid heart action in certain heart rhythm disorders.

The mechanism by which this ancient drug improves the heartbeat has been unknown for centuries, but recent research has begun to unravel the mystery. During each of the electrical impulses which drive the heart, sodium ion flows in across the cell wall for a brief period, and after the electrical impulse the heart cell must then recover its ionic balance in order to receive the next impulse. To accomplish this recovery, the cell has a "pump," an enzyme located within the cell wall, which uses energy to drive the sodium ion back out of the cell. There is now strong evidence that digitalis binds directly to this enzyme in the cell wall and interferes with its activity. By mechanisms that are still not fully understood, this interference with sodium pumping appears to make more calcium available within the cell. This, in turn, appears to cause more chemical sites on the protein filaments to attach to one another, increasing the force of heart contraction and partially overcoming the heart muscle failure.

With measures such as limitation of activity, restriction of salt intake, use of diuretics and digitalis, patients with disease of the heart muscle often can have many years of relatively comfortable existence.

Prevention of Heart Failure

As research begins to uncover the fundamental defects in the heart muscle cell that cause it to fail, it seems possible that new medications will be developed that can specifically correct such defects. However, even more hopeful is the increased research activity being directed toward preventing heart disease and heart failure. Two types of disease, high blood pressure and atherosclerosis, deserve special mention in this connection since they are in certain ways related, and since they are at the very top of the list of killers in Western societies.

It is now well-established that the higher the blood pressure, the greater the risk of developing atherosclerosis prematurely. This may be due to an effect of the elevated blood pressure in hastening the deposition of cholesterol and other fats directly into the walls of the arteries. Whatever the mechanism, patients with high blood pressure clearly have an increased risk of dying from coronary heart disease and heart attack, as well as from atherosclerotic disease of the blood vessels to the brain, which leads to stroke. The great advances in recent years in developing effective new drugs for lowering the blood pressure appear likely to reverse, at least in part, this toll from high blood pressure. Thus, if the blood pressure can be lowered and maintained in a normal range by drug administration, the risk of dying from stroke and other complications can be reduced. Even more importantly, if the high blood pressure is detected and treated early in its course, it is even possible that the more rapid development of atherosclerosis will be prevented.

Most important of all is the problem of atherosclerosis itself, and the "epidemic" of heart attacks that are a result of it. The possibility exists that measures can be taken to prevent the development of atherosclerosis in the coronary arteries, or actually to reverse the process once it has begun. Within the next few years we will see a great deal of research sponsored by the National Heart and Lung Institute of the National Institutes of Health designed to answer the following two questions:

1 Will diet and other treatment aimed at lowering the cholesterol and triglyceride blood levels in patients with established atherosclerosis *reverse* the trend toward early death from heart attack?

2 Will early dieting and/or drug treatment to lower blood lipid levels *prevent* the development of atherosclerosis in individuals who are found to have elevated blood lipid levels early in life?

The answers to these two questions remain uncertain at present, and there also are a number of patients who develop heart attack or stroke who do *not* have elevated levels of cholesterol or triglycerides in the bloodstream. In such patients, the role of diabetes, and obesity, as well as genetic constitution, will need further study relative to possible preventive measures.

Therefore, in the coming years a major focus for research will be on preventing heart disease and heart failure, as well as on halting or reversing the damaging effects of various diseases on the heart muscle itself. In the case of high blood pressure that is detected and treated, and in individuals with serious valvular heart disease who undergo corrective surgery, we are well on the way to preventing the long-standing wear and tear on the heart muscle that in the past have led to end-stage heart failure.

REFERENCES

General

1973 Heart Facts (E. M. 609A), American Heart Association, New York, 1973 (pamphlet).

Scientific Works

Braunwald, E., Ross, J., Jr., and Sonnenblick, E. H., *Mechanisms of Contraction of the Normal and Failing Heart*, 2d ed., Little Brown and Company, Boston, 1975.

Fowler, N. O., "Differential Diagnosis of Cardiomyopathies," *Progress in Cardiovascular Disease*, **14**:113, 1971.

Goodwin, J. F., "Clarification of the Cardiomyopathies," *Modern Concepts of Cardiovascular Disease*, **41**:41, 1972.

Spann, J. F., Mason, D. T., and Zelis, R. F., "Recent Advances in the Understanding of Heart Failure," *Modern Concepts of Cardiovascular Disease*, **39**:79, 1970.

Chapter 10

Inborn Heart Disease

Abnormalities of the heart that are inborn (present at birth) are referred to as "congenital" heart disease. This occurs in about eight out of every thousand births. In some cases, the defect is slight; in other instances, a minimal defect at birth may become progressively more severe during later life. Most often, however, an abnormal heart sound or murmur is heard or blueness of the skin ("cyanosis") is noted in the newborn period, or in early childhood, and occasionally congenital heart disease is discovered for the first time in the adult. Many complex and unusual types of congenital heart disease are now well known, and most of these can now be treated by operation thanks to advances in modern surgical techniques (Chapter 11). Thus, the child born with a congenital heart defect has a far better chance of survival today than 15 or even 10 years ago. Among these many types of defects, only a few of the most common will be discussed below.

The cause of most congenital heart disease is unknown. A very small percentage of cases are known to be due to German measles occurring in the mother during early pregnancy, and some other cases also may be due to unrecognized infections or other factors occurring during pregnancy. Although a few congenital heart defects run in families, this is distinctly unusual, and there is little evidence at present for transmission of most congenital defects through the genes.

Frequently, cardiac catheterization and angiocardiography are performed whenever the diagnosis of congenital heart disease is suspected in order to determine whether or not the defect is of a type that can be repaired by operation. Sometimes, the cardiac catheterization test and consideration of surgery can be postponed until the child has been allowed to grow for several years. During this period there is now much less tendency among physicians to place severe restrictions on the child, since it has been found that in general he will limit his own activity. Therefore every effort is usually made to allow the child to lead as normal a life as possible. If necessary, surgical correction, or partial correction of some types of defects can be done at a very early age, but most corrective operations for congenital heart disease discovered in childhood are performed between the ages of five and twelve years.

Recently, some of the most important advances in the treatment of inborn heart disease have occurred in the management of the critically ill infant. This group of patients constitutes about one-third of all patients born with congenital heart disease. These infants usually have a severe form of one of the defects described below (or certain other more complex lesions) which result in either marked blueness (low oxygen content in the blood in the arteries) or severe heart failure. However, more than half of these lesions have now been found to be potentially amenable to complete repair. Therefore, current practice is to carry out a cardiac catheterization in the critically ill newborn infant and, whenever feasible, to immediately carry out an operation that will improve or correct the situation. When this vigorous approach is applied in pediatric heart centers, up to 65 percent of these infants have survived. The manner in which the precise diagnosis of these defects has evolved over the past few years has gone hand-in-hand with and has, in fact, helped to make possible some of the important technical advances in heart surgery. Perhaps the most significant diagnostic method has been cineangiocardiography, the exposure of high-speed x-ray motion pictures which provide a picture of injected liquid that is opaque to x-rays as it travels with the blood through the abnormal heart.

The most common types of congenital heart defects can be divided into four major groups:

I   Narrowing or constriction of a blood vessel or a heart valve
II Abnormal holes or communications
  A   An abnormal connection between two blood vessels (patent ductus)
  B   A hole in the muscle, or septum, that separates two chambers of the heart (ventricular or atrial septal defect)
III A combination of I and II, that is, both narrowing of a vessel and a septal defect
IV Abnormal connections of the blood vessels leading to or from the heart

The latter two types of defects may cause blueness of the skin (or cyanosis), the so-called blue baby. A brief description of several of the commonest types of congenital heart disease within each of these major subgroups follows.

Narrowing or Constriction of a Blood Vessel or Heart Valve

Narrowing (Coarctation) of the Aorta   In this condition, there is a short area of narrowing of the large artery that leads from the left-sided pumping chamber of the heart. Therefore, the lesion is not strictly a congenital *heart* defect, since it is located a considerable distance away from the heart, beyond the branches of the aorta that supply blood to the head and arms (Figure 10-1*B*). The severe narrowing causes the blood pressure to be elevated in the arms, and it may be impossible to obtain a blood pressure in the legs using the blood pressure cuff. This blood pressure difference between the arms and legs usually is the clue to the diagnosis of this disorder. The high pressure in the aorta puts an added strain on the heart, and other problems may occur such as pain in the legs due to insufficient blood flow. More seriously, the high blood pressure may become progressively more severe and, if the problem is not recognized, rupture of a blood vessel in the brain or other serious complications can ensue.

The results of operation for coarctation of the aorta have been very successful. The procedure generally is performed in childhood and usually consists of cutting out the narrowed area and reattaching the aorta to itself to give a channel of normal diameter. The operation is carried out without opening the heart itself.

Congenital Aortic Stenosis (Aortic Valve Narrowing)   Aortic stenosis in the adult already has been discussed in Chapter 5. In childhood, however, the usual cause for severe aortic valve narrowing is not rheumatic fever, but a congenital deformity of the aortic valve. Often there are only two leaflets of the valve, rather than the normal three, and they are partially fused together. It is now considered likely that mild forms of this two-leaflet aortic valve, which may not even be detected in childhood, are responsible for a considerable number of cases of aortic stenosis seen in adulthood. The abnormal valve motion results in time in scarring and narrowing of the opening. Unusual forms of congenital aortic stenosis also sometimes occur, areas of severe narrowing being found just below or above a normally formed aortic valve.

If the narrowing of the valve is very severe in childhood (proven by cardiac catheterization) an operation is undertaken regardless of age since there is some risk of the patient dying suddenly and unexpectedly. Also, symptoms can occur which are like those in the adult. The surgeon performs an open-heart operation, using the heart-lung machine, and directly examines the valve. Usually, in congenital aortic stenosis the surgeon can then open up the areas of the valve that adhere together, and generally a satisfactory opening is obtained without damaging the valve leaflets. Other unusual sites for the narrowing above or below also can usually be repaired surgically.

ATRIAL & VENTRICULAR SEPTAL DEFECTS

PATENT DUCTUS ARTERIOSUS & COARCTATION OF AORTA

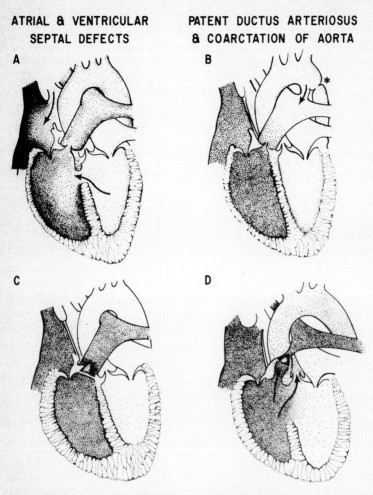

PULMONARY VALVE STENOSIS   PULMONARY STENOSIS & VSD

Figure 10-1 Common congenital or inborn heart defects.
Panel A: In ventricular septal defect there is a hole in the partition between the two pumping chambers of the heart, and blood is shunted from the left-sided pumping chamber (high pressure) into the right ventricle (lower arrow). In the same diagram, a hole between the two receiving chambers which also causes a shunt of red blood into the right side of the heart, is shown (upper arrow). The darker stippling indicates blue, or venous, blood and the lighter stippled areas indicate red, oxygenated blood as it mixes with

Pulmonic Stenosis (Pulmonic Valve Narrowing) The pulmonic valve normally opens wide when the right ventricle
contracts, allowing blood to be ejected freely into the pulmonary
artery and thence to the lungs. In one of the most common
congenital heart defects, there is failure of this valve to develop
normally, and the leaflets are fused together leaving only a small
opening. Therefore, the right-sided pumping chamber (right ventricle) is forced to develop a very high pressure in order to pump
blood across the narrowed valve. Usually there is a loud noise, or
murmur, as the blood is forced through the narrow orifice (Figure
10-1C). Sometimes, the narrowing occurs below a normal pulmonic valve, and in rare instances the narrowing is located in the
pulmonary artery, above the pulmonic valve. The consequences
of pulmonic valve narrowing are due to the strain placed on the
right ventricle which eventually may cause right-sided heart
failure.

As with aortic stenosis, usually it is possible for the valve to
be repaired by open heart surgery. The fused areas are divided to
relieve the obstruction. A comparison of the anatomy of the
aortic and pulmonic valves, however, shows that the coronary
arteries are near the aortic valve. In addition, the pulmonic valve
is subjected to much lower pressures, and some leakage can be

---

the venous blood. Although shown in the same diagram, these two defects
usually do not occur together.
Panel B: An abnormal channel between the aorta and the pulmonary artery is
shown at the arrow (patent ductus arteriosus). This lesion results in an
abnormal shunt of red blood from the aorta into the pulmonary artery and
through the lungs. Although usually not occurring in the same patient, a
narrowing of the aorta is shown at the asterisk (coarctation of the aorta).
Panel C: Inborn, or congenital, narrowing of the pulmonic valve (pulmonary
valve stenosis). This lesion results in marked overwork of the right ventricle
because it must develop a high pressure to force blood across the narrowed
valve. The flow of blue and red blood through the heart is otherwise normal,
since there are no holes between the heart chambers.
Panel D: A combination of inborn defects commonly seen in "blue babies":
both pulmonary stenosis and a ventricular septal defect are present
(tetralogy of Fallot). In this case, the high pressure developed by the right
ventricle because of the narrowed pulmonary valve causes blue blood to be
shunted across the ventricular septal defect in an opposite direction from
that shown in Panel A. Consequently, blue venous blood mixes with red
blood on the left side of the heart and the patient is blue, or cyanotic.

well-tolerated. For these reasons, the operation for pulmonic stenosis is less difficult and somewhat safer than that for aortic stenosis. The operation is generally performed in childhood, although the defect is compatible with survival to adulthood, and many adults have undergone successful operations for congenital pulmonic stenosis.

Abnormal Holes or Communications in the Heart

A Connection between the Aorta and the Pulmonary Artery (Patent Ductus Arteriosus)   Every baby prior to birth has a short channel connecting the aorta and the pulmonary artery (Figure 10-1*B*). Since the lungs are not used, this channel allows blood pumped by the fetal heart to bypass the lungs. Normally, within a few hours or days after birth this channel closes. In a common form of congenital heart disease (which does not really involve a *heart* defect), this channel remains open indefinitely.

As discussed in Chapter 1, the normal pressure in the aorta is about 5 times higher than that in the pulmonary artery. Therefore, it can be understood how blood would readily flow across this short channel from the aorta to the pulmonary artery, sending excess blood that has already been oxygenated through the lungs. When the channel of the patent ductus is large, this so-called *shunt* may actually produce failure of the left-sided pumping chamber. Thus, this chamber must pump the normal quantity of blood, together with that which runs back from the aorta to the pulmonary artery and thence back to the left ventricle in a short circuit. A typical heart murmur is generally present, a cardiac catheterization shows the presence of an abnormally high content of oxygen in a sample of blood obtained from the pulmonary artery, and an angiogram clearly shows the abnormal channel.

One of the earliest successful operations on the circulation within the chest was the correction of a patent ductus arteriosus. It is not necessary to use the heart-lung machine because sutures can be placed directly through the abnormal channel to close it. This procedure, which is not truly a heart operation, can be carried out very safely and the results have been highly satisfactory.

A Hole between the Two Pumping Chambers (Ventricular Septal Defect)   When an abnormal hole exists between the two pumping chambers (the left and right ventricles) blood flows through the hole into the right ventricle because pressure is lower than in the left ventricle. Thus, there is an abnormal "shunt" of blood, and since the left ventricle must pump blood both to the body as well as through the hole, it is overburdened (Figure 10-1*B*). In addition, the excessive flow of oxygenated blood through the lungs can be associated with an abnormally high pressure in the pulmonary artery. Eventually, the small blood vessels in the lungs may be damaged by the excess blood flow and high pressure (as is also the case with a large patent ductus, see above).

The operation for correction of ventricular septal defect usually is carried out in childhood. Using the heart-lung machine, an incision is made through the wall of the right-sided pumping chamber (right ventricle), and a patch of woven plastic material is sewn in place to cover the hole, thereby abolishing the blood shunt. A few ventricular septal defects, particularly small ones, close spontaneously during early childhood. (This is possibly the only congenital heart defect which is "outgrown.")

A Hole between the Two Receiving Chambers (Atrial Septal Defect)   As shown in Figure 10-1*A*, when there is an abnormal hole in the partition between the left atrium and the right atrium, red oxygenated blood tends to flow across the defect into the right atrium creating an abnormal shunt of blood. The right-sided pumping chamber (right ventricle) must then pump the normal amount of blood through the lungs, together with the excess blood from the shunt. In addition, as with ventricular septal defect, the excessive flow of blood through the lungs and a high pressure in the pulmonary artery eventually may result in damage to the small blood vessels within the lungs.

Generally, the heart murmur with an atrial defect is difficult to hear, and in many patients symptoms do not occur until adulthood. The operation for this defect, which requires use of the heart-lung machine, consists of placing a plastic patch over the hole, or sometimes sewing shut the edges of the hole directly.

Ventricular Septal Defect and Pulmonic Valve Narrowing (Tetralogy of Fallot)

Most "blue babies" who survive infancy, as well as older individuals with blueness of the skin (cyanosis) which is due to congenital heart disease, have this combination of lesions named after the French anatomist Fallot who described the defect in 1888 from autopsy specimens. The history of the first operation for blue babies constitutes an exciting chapter in the development of modern heart surgery, and the reason that the operation works may be understood by referring to Figure 10-1D. When there is narrowing of the pulmonic valve (or of the zone immediately beneath the pulmonic valve, as is frequently the case), the right-sided pumping chamber must develop a high pressure in order to force blood across the valve and through the lungs; however, if the narrowing of the pulmonic valve *and* a hole in the partition between the pumping chambers (ventricular septal defect) are both present, less blood can be forced across the narrowed valve. This is so because the hole in the partition between the pumping chambers serves to "decompress" the right ventricle and allows part of the blue venous blood returning to the right side of the heart from the body to be shunted across into the left ventricle and out the aorta (see diagram). Two effects ensue: First, this blue blood mixes in the left ventricle with red blood returning from the lungs and is pumped out into the aorta. Secondly, the amount of blood that enters the pulmonary artery and the lungs is greatly reduced, which results in an abnormally small return of red, oxygenated blood reaching the left ventricle in the first place (diagram). Since only a small amount of red blood mixes with blue blood crossing from the right ventricle, *most* of the blood pumped into the aorta and to the body by the left ventricle is blue and the patient shows very severe cyanosis or blueness. This can result in spells of unconsciousness, marked limitation of activity, and difficulties with blood clots.

The surgical approach devised in 1944 by Drs. Alfred Blalock (a surgeon) and Helen Taussig (a pediatric cardiologist) of The Johns Hopkins Hospital was beautifully simple, and became the first successful "blue-baby operation." It was devised before the development of a workable heart-lung machine, and before the possibility was ever considered that total repair of the disorder might become possible. It was surmised that if the amount of blood flow through the lungs could be improved in some manner, the proportion of oxygenated blood mixing with blue blood in the left ventricle would result in a relatively higher oxygen content per unit of blood, and thereby diminish the cyanosis. Their solution was to create an *artificial* patent ductus arteriosus (see above). That is, from within the chest one end of an artery that normally supplies the arm was detached leaving the near end of the artery normally attached to the aorta (this does not result in damage to the arm). The cut end was then sutured to the pulmonary artery, creating an artificial channel to that vessel. Since the pressure in the pulmonary artery beyond the narrowed pulmonic valve was far lower than in the aorta, blood flowed continuously from the aorta through the newly attached segment of the artery to the lungs where it was oxygenated. It then flowed to the left-sided pumping chamber to be pumped to the body.

The results were dramatic. Most blue babies receiving this operation became pink almost immediately, while still in the operating room, and they subsequently had a number of years of satisfactory existence. With time, many of these children outgrew the effects of the operation; that is, the size of the artificial shunt became too small for the needs of the body as the child grew. Many of these patients have now undergone total correction of the narrowed area in the right ventricle and pulmonic valve, together with closure of the hole in the ventricular septum. The Blalock-Taussig operation, as it is now known, and variations of it are still performed in very young children and infants in whom severe cyanosis is present. In older children it is now usually preferable to undertake complete repair of the two defects.

Abnormal Connections of the Large Blood Vessels Leading to or from the Heart

Another common cause of the blue baby is a severe congenital defect which usually results in early death if the infant is untreated. This condition, called "transposition of the great arteries" (great arteries referring to the aorta and pulmonary artery), consists of complete reversal of the attachments of two large vessels coming from the heart. Thus, the aorta arises from the *right*-sided pumping chamber (and therefore receives blue blood from the veins of the body) and the pulmonary artery arises from the *left*-sided pumping chamber. This means that the left ventricle simply pumps oxygenated red blood around and around through the lungs and back to itself in a circle, whereas the right ventricle pumps blue venous blood to the body. Of course, some mixing of blue and red blood *must* occur within the heart in order for the infant to survive at all, and the lesion is associated with either a hole between the receiving chambers (atrial septal defect) or between the pumping chambers (ventricular septal defect). A complex operation for the complete correction of this defect that consists of rearranging the large veins that bring blood into the heart from the body and the lungs has been successfully applied in recent years. However, the operation generally is not feasible in newborn infants. Temporary treatment for such newborn infants has been provided by a procedure which allows the creation or enlargement of a hole between the two receiving chambers during the course of a cardiac catheterization. A balloon positioned at the tip of a catheter is inflated and then pulled rapidly across the partition between the left atrium and the right atrium, thereby enlarging the hole and allowing better mixing of red and blue blood between these two receiving chambers. When this procedure is successful, it has often been possible for the infant to survive and grow to a size large enough to allow complete correction of this defect.

All together, about 80 percent of the congenital heart defects which are compatible with early survival of the infant can now be corrected surgically in a satisfactory manner.

REFERENCES

General

A Guide for Teachers. Children with Heart Disease (E. M. 25), American Heart Association, New York, 1971 (pamphlet).
If Your Child Has Congenital Heart Disease (E. M. 250), American Heart Association, New York, 1970 (pamphlet).

1973 Heart Facts (E. M. 509*A*), American Heart Association, New York, 1973 (pamphlet).

Scientific Works

Danilowicz, D. A., and Ross, J., Jr., "Congenital Heart Disease," in *Cardiac and Vascular Diseases* by H. L. Conn, Jr., and O. Horowitz (eds.), Lea and Febiger, Philadelphia, 1971, p. 619.

Talner, N. S., and Campbell, A. G. M., "Recognition and Management of Cardiologic Problems in the Newborn Infant," *Progress in Cardiovascular Disease*, **15:**159, 1972.

Heart Surgery

Early Attempts at Heart Surgery

In 1882 the great German surgeon Theodore Billroth stated: "Let no surgeon who wishes to preserve the respect of his colleagues ever attempt to suture the heart." Nevertheless, by 1895 several attempts to repair stab wounds to the human heart had been made in Norway and in Italy, and in 1896 Ludwig Rehn of Frankfurt, Germany, finally was successful, repairing a laceration of the heart in a patient who had sustained a wound during a brawl. Although it was not until after World War II that elective operations for repairing damaged heart valves became regularly successful, in a few remarkable isolated attempts, patients survived pioneering early operations. Probably the first was that by Theodore Tuffier, a French surgeon who earlier had successfully removed a portion of the lung for tuberculosis. He performed the first heart-valve operation in 1912 when he operated upon a young

man with narrowing of the aortic valve, and by pressing inward
on the wall of the aorta near the valve succeeded in stretching the
valve tissue. The patient, remarkably enough, survived and was
improved for several years. Narrowing of the mitral valve (mitral
stenosis) was an extremely common cardiac condition at that
time and was a cause of death in many young patients suffering
from rheumatic fever and subsequent scarring of the valves.
There had been much interest in developing experimental methods for opening the scarred mitral valve, and in the 1920s there
were a number of efforts, and a few rare successes, at the surgical
alleviation of this condition. As early as 1923 Elliot Cutler of
Boston operated on an eleven-year-old girl for mitral stenosis
using a knife-like instrument inserted through the left ventricle to
cut the scarred, adherent leaflets. The patient lived $4^{1}/_{2}$ years and
was somewhat improved. In his other attempts, however, the
operation was unsuccessful and the patients died. In 1925 in
London, surgeon Henry Souttar operated on a child with leakage
and narrowing of the mitral valve. He used an approach that was
to prove successful more than twenty years later, inserting his
finger through the receiving chamber (the left atrium) and dividing the adhesions of the valve. This patient survived and had
lessened symptoms for several years; operations by others were
attempted at about the same time without success. In the late
1930s Gordon Murray, a Canadian surgeon, had several successes
with inserting a "sling" constructed of a length of vein in order to
reinforce a portion of the leaking mitral valve; this operation was
far ahead of its time. In 1937 Robert Gross of Boston successfully
repaired a patent ductus arteriosus without complication, thereby
performing perhaps the first "curative" heart operation, although
this operation is not directly on the heart, since it involves closing
an abnormal communication between the pulmonary artery and
the aorta (see Chapter 10).

Following the many medical advances which accompanied
World War II (blood transfusion, the development of antibiotics,
and perfection of anesthetic techniques), several American surgeons almost simultaneously began to have success with the
operation for mitral stenosis. In 1948 Horace Smithy of Charles-
ton, using a knife-like instrument to remove a portion of the

mitral valve, was successful in a twenty-one-year-old woman, although subsequently she developed heart failure and lived less than a year; several of his later patients survived, however. Also in 1948 Dwight Harkin of Boston was successful in restoring mobility of the mitral valve by cutting out a portion of the valve tissue, and in the same year Charles Bailey of Philadelphia and Sir Russell Brock of London had success using Souttar's technique, the index finger being fitted with a small curved knife blade to split open the adherent valve leaflets. The modern era of cardiac surgery had begun.

This type of procedure, and others in which the heart is not opened and emptied of blood, often are termed "closed-heart surgery." During such operations the heart beats normally and supports the circulation. However, most surgical procedures on the heart are now performed with the benefit of direct vision while the heart is opened. This, of course, requires some other means of supporting the circulation while the operation is in progress. The development of such artificial circulatory support systems, commonly called "heart-lung machines," constituted an important chapter in the development of modern heart surgery.

Heart-Lung Machines

Early attempts to support the circulation in order to allow direct access to the heart were made using "cross circulation" between the patient and a normal subject, generally a member of the patient's own family. By connecting tubing to an artery and vein, the "donor" was attached to the "recipient," the patient undergoing the operation. This procedure, however, was soon found to result in some risk to the donor as well as considerable difficulties in controlling the amount of the cross circulation. A better approach was necessary.

In 1953 John Gibbon of Philadelphia, culminating years of experimental work on the development of an artificial circulatory support system, carried out the first successful perfusion using a man-made oxygenator (lung) and pump. The eighteen-year-old patient had an atrial septal defect (hole between the receiving chambers) which was closed in the operation, and the patient recovered after thirty minutes of artificial support. This early machine employed wire-mesh screens to spread the blood in an atmosphere of oxygen and was followed by many other types of heart-lung machines developed during the 1950s. All of them, however, consist basically of two components: the oxygenator, which accepts the dark venous blood coming from the patient and by exposure to an oxygen-gas mixture removes the carbon dioxide and replaces the oxygen, and a pump, which replaces the function of the patient's own heart.

In order to empty the heart and put it at rest, it is necessary to "bypass" the heart and lungs by diverting the blue blood returning to the heart through tubes which carry it into the heart-lung machine. A large surface area for blood gas exchange is created within the machine, and the oxygenated blood then passes to a pump which returns it to an artery of the patient. The oxygenator may consist of a filming device using screens or moving disks, or a foaming device in which small bubbles of oxygen are passed through the blood to provide a large surface area for gas exchange; the bubbles are then removed. A newer development is the so-called membrane oxygenator in which, as in the lung, the blood does not come into direct contact with the oxygen atmosphere but rather is passed within a series of thin plastic films which allow exchange of oxygen and carbon dioxide. The pumps in early machines resembled piston pumps, like those used for pumping industrial fluids. At the present time so-called roller pumps often are used in which plastic or rubber tubing is gently milked by rotating arms fitted with rollers, a method that has a much less damaging effect on the elements of the blood. Generally, the heart is stopped, or "arrested," and cooled during the operation, and often the metabolic needs of the whole body also are lowered by cooling the blood during the period of support. The heart-lung machine has now come into routine use. It has many safety features, and its use in a modern cardiovascular center carries very little risk, while making possible many types of complex operations within the heart.

Valve Replacement

Successful clinical use of the pump oxygenator for total heart-lung bypass opened a new era in the surgical treatment of heart disease. However, surgical therapy of acquired valvular heart disease remained seriously limited by the far-advanced deterioration of these valves. Thickening, distortion, and calcification of valve leaflets usually prevented the successful restoration of valve function except in some patients with mitral stenosis. Even in cases which appeared suitable for various surgical techniques of repairing valve leaflets, long-term results were disappointing. The necessity for valve replacement in such patients soon became obvious.

Early attempts at artificial replacement of cardiac valves consisted of the use of flexible leaflets constructed from a variety of synthetic materials to substitute for one, two, or all three leaflets of the aortic valve. Despite original enthusiasm for such techniques, subsequent fatigue and tearing of the leaflets or narrowing of the valve due to tissue overgrowth demonstrated the need for an artificial valve (prosthesis) which did not depend on flexible synthetic leaflets. Designs for such a prosthesis, the "caged-ball valve," had been available for more than a century. This prosthetic valve consists of a metal ring base for sewing into the heart at the appropriate valve site, three or more curved metal struts originating at the base and extending 1/2 to 3/4 inch in the direction of blood flow, and a silicone or metallic ball (poppet), which moves between the metal base and the curved ends of the metal struts. When this artificial valve is in the closed position, the ball, or poppet, sits in the metal ring base and no blood flows through it. The ball moves from the ring base to the apex of the cage as blood flows through it during systole (ventricular contraction) in the aortic valve prosthesis and during diastole (ventricular filling) in the mitral valve prosthesis (Figure 11-1).

The caged-ball principle was first utilized by Charles Hufnagel of Washington, D.C., who designed an aortic valve prosthesis which he inserted as early as 1951 in the aorta quite distant from the heart for the treatment of severe leakage of the aortic valve. Dwight Harkin of Boston in 1960 reported the first clinical use of a caged-ball artificial aortic valve placed directly in the position of the natural aortic valve. It remained, however, for surgeon Albert Starr and M. Lowell Edwards of Portland, Oregon, to refine and apply on a wide scale a caged-ball cardiac valve prosthesis, first for mitral valve replacement and subsequently for aortic valve replacement. Clinical experience with the

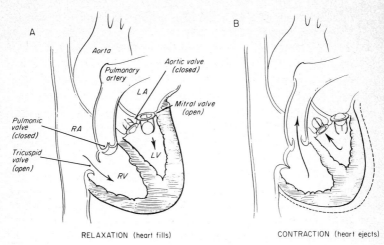

A

Aorta

Pulmonary
artery

Aortic valve
(closed)

LA

Mitral valve
(open)

Pulmonic
valve
(closed)

RA

Tricuspid
valve
(open)

LV

RV

B

RELAXATION (heart fills)

CONTRACTION (heart ejects)

Figure 11-1 Artificial heart valves placed in the aortic and mitral positions. The caged-ball valve prostheses are shown in operation as the heart relaxes and contracts. In *Panel A*, the heart is relaxed and the mitral ball-valve prosthesis is open, allowing flow of blood from the left-sided receiving chamber (the left atrium, LA) into the left ventricle.

In *Panel B*, during heart contraction the aortic ball valve opens to allow ejection of blood into the aorta, and the ball in the mitral valve prosthesis moves to the closed position, preventing backward flow of blood from the pumping chamber into the left atrium.

The valves on the right side of the heart (pulmonic and tricuspid) are functioning normally.

Starr-Edwards artificial valves soon became widespread, and effective surgical therapy was applied to increasing numbers of patients with acquired valvular heart disease. Subsequent modifications in design of the caged-ball prostheses made their insertion easier and improved the effect of valve replacement in reversing the signs and symptoms of cardiac disease. More recently, smaller prostheses utilizing either a tilting disk or a disk moving within a small cage have been developed in an attempt to decrease the amount of artificial material protruding into the left ventricular cavity in patients requiring a mitral valve prosthesis. At the time of operation the surgeon removes the thickened, distorted, and often calcified diseased valve and then inserts the prosthetic valve sewing its metal ring base into the site of the previous valve (Figure 11-1).

A major problem with the use of artificial cardiac valves is the tendency for clot formation to occur on the metal surfaces which constitute the base of the valve and/or its struts. This clot formation may either interfere with the normal movement of the prosthetic valve or may break off, circulate through the blood-stream, and occlude small arteries to various organs such as the brain, kidney, and spleen. For this reason, the majority of patients with artificial heart valves have been treated with blood-thinning agents (anticoagulants) to prevent this tendency for clot formation. Other approaches to this clotting problem have been the use of fabric-covered artificial heart valves and the use of homografts or heterografts for valve replacement. The former consists of a caged-ball valve with a thin layer of cloth covering the metal base and the metal struts. The areas of cloth covering became encapsulated by normal tissue within two or three months following insertion, and the tendency for clot formation on a metal surface therefore is reduced. "Homograft valves" consist of human valve leaflets which are obtained from the donor at the time of a sterile autopsy. Homografts are treated with a preservative, frozen, and later inserted in the patient (recipient) at the time of valve replacement. "Heterografts" are valve leaflets obtained from another species (for example, swine); they also have been used successfully as a substitute for scarred, nonmobile valves in patients with rheumatic heart disease. The incidence of clot formation in patients with homograft or hetero-graft valves is negligible. However, these valves have been in use for a shorter period of time than the caged-ball valve prosthesis and the long-term results of their use are still unknown.

Surgery for Congenital Heart Disease

Great strides have been made in the field of congenital heart disease since the introduction of the pump oxygenator. There are now few inborn heart conditions which cannot be either correct-ed or ameliorated by surgery (see Chapter 10). Commonly performed operative procedures include the closure of a defect between the left and right pumping chambers of the heart (ventricular septal defect), the suture or patch closure of a hole between the left and right receiving chambers (atrial septal defect), and the opening of a narrowed pulmonic valve (pulmonic stenosis). The "shunting" procedures devised by Drs. Blalock, Taussig, and others, which divert blue blood through the lungs, permit infants born with complex abnormal cardiac anatomy and inadequate oxygen in the systemic arterial blood ("blue baby") to survive to an age where definitive surgical correction may be performed. Recently, many new surgical techniques have been devised for the complete correction of a variety of complex congenital cardiac defects. For example, complete surgical repair of the most common type of cyanotic (blue) heart disease, tetralogy of Fallot (ventricular septal defect and pulmonic stenosis) is now commonplace. In this operation the narrowed area between the right ventricular and pulmonary artery is opened and the ventricular septal defect closed. Refinements in heart-lung bypass techniques have enabled corrective operative techniques to be offered to children in the first year of life.

Surgery of Coronary Artery Disease

Coronary artery disease, which can decrease coronary blood flow to the heart muscle, is the principal cause of death among the adult population of the United States.

In 1935, the surgeon Claude Beck attempted to increase coronary blood flow in a patient with coronary artery disease by creating adhesions between the outer layer of the left ventricular cardiac muscle (epicardium) and the heart's outer blood vessel-containing sac, the pericardium. Beck induced cardiac-pericardial communications by scraping the epicardium and pericardium with a mechanical burr. Epicardial abrasion was also obtained using talc, sand, and asbestos. But the scar tissue which later formed terminated the growth of the new blood vessel connections between pericardium and cardiac muscle, and few patients benefited symptomatically. A major advance in coronary artery surgery took place in 1946 when Arthur Vineberg, a Canadian surgeon, demonstrated experimentally that a systemic artery bleeding freely from side branches could be implanted into the heart muscle. Vineberg demonstrated that definite connections formed following operation between the implanted artery and the coronary circulation. Later he reported clinical applications of this method and well-documented evidence obtained at autopsies showing that increased blood flow to cardiac muscle ("myocardial revascularization") was accomplished by internal mammary artery implantation. However, the increase in myocardial blood flow following internal mammary artery implantation is small, and many patients developed a heart attack during surgery or in the immediate post-operative period.

The first successful direct coronary artery surgery was reported by Charles Bailey of Philadelphia in 1957. Two of his three patients operated on for the removal of obstructive lesions in the right coronary artery survived. However, subsequent experience revealed that direct surgery on lesions in the major coronary arteries is often unsuccessful and is associated with a high risk of heart attack and death. Disappointment with the direct surgical attack on occluded coronary arteries led Rene Favaloro in Cleveland to extensively apply use of the vein bypass graft to channel blood from the aorta to the right coronary artery in 1967. Subsequently, there has been widespread use of this technique throughout the world to treat patients with symptoms from coronary artery disease. At the start of the operation, a long surface vein is taken from one leg and cut in appropriate lengths to be used for aortocoronary artery vein bypass grafts. As many as four or five such vein grafts may be employed in a patient with atherosclerotic disease involving several major branches of the right and left coronary arteries (Figure 11-2).

The introduction in 1958 by F. Mason Sones of selective coronary angiography proved to be an essential step in the preoperative and postoperative evaluation of patients with coronary artery disease. Cardiac catheterization and coronary angiography are necessary for the preoperative evaluation of all candidates for coronary artery surgery. Obviously, for vein bypass graft operations to be feasible, there must be open coronary arteries *beyond* the areas of artery narrowing, into which the vein bypass graft can be implanted.

Although the initial results of coronary artery bypass graft surgery have been encouraging, with 60 to 80 percent of patients

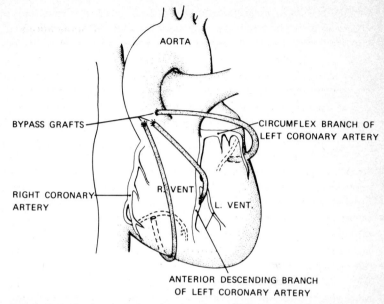

AORTA

BYPASS GRAFTS

CIRCUMFLEX BRANCH OF
LEFT CORONARY ARTERY

RIGHT CORONARY
ARTERY

R. VENT

L. VENT.

ANTERIOR DESCENDING BRANCH
OF LEFT CORONARY ARTERY

Figure 11-2 In the examples shown, vein grafts have been placed from the aorta to all three major branches of the cornary arteries supplying the heart. The grafts are attached beyond a site of narrowing or obstruction in the coronary artery, allowing blood to "bypass" the narrowed zone. Sometimes only one or two grafts, or as many as five grafts are used.

relieved of their chest pain, the long-term results of coronary artery surgery and its effect on the natural history of coronary artery disease is uncertain. In addition, the current indications for coronary artery surgery remain controversial.

Patients with coronary artery disease and a previous heart attack often develop heart failure. In many patients this is due to a discrete area of destroyed heart muscle which has been replaced by scar tissue forming an area of the left ventricle which does not participate in cardiac contraction. The surgical removal of this area of scar tissue in patients with coronary artery disease and severe heart failure has sometimes proved to be successful in relieving symptoms due to heart failure. Additional complications of a heart attack which may require cardiac surgery result from diminished coronary blood flow to the papillary muscles support-ing the mitral valve or to the muscle partition (septum) between the ventricles. Acute or chronic mitral valve leakage resulting from involvement of one or both the papillary muscles at the time of a heart attack may necessitate mitral valve replacement. Also, a ruptured ventricular septum due to damage from a heart attack may require surgical closure in order for the patient to survive.

Heart Transplantation

Whether or not cardiac transplantation eventually becomes a standard method in the treatment of heart disease, the direct demonstration of its technical feasibility in human beings by Christian Barnard in 1967 was certainly a "first" in cardiac surgical practice. The laboratory endeavors leading up to this feat were initiated by Carrell and Guthrie in 1905, who implanted a heart into the neck of a dog, and by the Russian Demikhov who performed the first experimental cardiac transplant in which the heart was sutured into its normal position. Norman Shumway and his colleagues at Stanford Medical Center in California developed many of the operative techniques now used and studied the immunologic responses invoked by the transplanted heart. Be-cause of public awareness of this unique surgical procedure and the sensationalism that has distorted its objective assessment, the reception of transplantation has oscillated markedly between enthusiasm and disillusion.

Patients with end-stage heart failure from diseases involving the heart muscle, including severe generalized coronary artery disease, have formed the majority of patients undergoing heart transplantation. The donor preferably is a young and otherwise healthy individual who has died abruptly. This qualification limits donors to the victims of accidents involving severe head injuries, or to those dying from irreversible stroke or brain tumor. Objective criteria of death must be obtained, such as cessation of spontaneous respiration and absence of electrical activity of the brain. Once it is decided that the donor is beyond hope of recovery, supportive measures designed to preserve the viability and function of the heart itself are instituted.

Prior to heart transplantation, red blood cells, white blood cells, and tissue samples from the donor and the patient who will receive the heart transplant (recipient) are evaluated for tissue compatibility in the laboratory in order to decrease the likelihood of immunologic rejection of the transplanted heart through the development of antibodies by the recipient against the foreign heart tissue. Measures to prevent this immunologic response to heart transplantation are mandatory during the pre- and postoperative period in order for heart transplantation to be successful. Blood A, B, O typing with compatibility between donor and recipient in white blood cells also is necessary.

The surgical technique for transplantation of the heart employs procedures regularly used in other cardiac surgical operations. After brain death occurs, the donor heart is maintained in the donor's chest cavity until the recipient has been supported on a heart-lung bypass machine and his diseased heart removed. This is accomplished by dividing the aorta and pulmonary artery and by removing part of the atria (receiving chambers) (see Figure 11-1). The back portion of the recipient's atria with attached large veins (venae cavae) and pulmonary veins remain in place, permitting ready surgical attachment of the donor atria by suturing. The subsequent attachment by sutures of the donor's pulmonary artery and aorta to the cut ends of the recipient's vessels completes the insertion of the new heart.

The development of high blood-antibody levels during the first four weeks after transplantation may lead to an early rejection of the transplanted heart by the recipient, or late rejection may occur several months or years after transplantation. The rejection process initially involves antigen-antibody reactions leading to small blood vessel damage and cardiac tissue inflammation. The clinical signals of heart rejection include weakness, signs of heart failure, inflammation of the pericardium, changes in the electrocardiogram, and an elevation in serum enzymes due to their release into the bloodstream from the damaged heart muscle.

Following the operation, drugs which decrease antibody formation ("immunosuppressive" drugs) are used in varying combinations to prevent rejection of the transplanted heart.

These medications, which have had variable success in the prevention of acute cardiac rejection, must be taken indefinitely by the patient following heart transplantation, and their dosage is increased when clinical signs of impending rejection become apparent. Unfortunately, they also reduce the patient's resistance to various infections.

There have been over 200 heart transplantations performed in the past six years, and the great majority of these patients have subsequently died due to cardiac rejection or infection. Curiously, extensive narrowing of previously normal coronary arteries in the donor heart has been observed in many of the patients dying one or more years following cardiac transplantation. As an example, survival statistics for the initial 47 patients undergoing heart transplantation at Stanford Medical Center showed a 40 percent survival at one year, 36 percent at two years, and a projected 17 percent three-year survival. In 25 patients who survived the initial three months following surgery, survival was 71 percent at one year, 65 percent at two years and 31 percent at three years. There has been a somewhat encouraging increase in the one-year survival after transplantation in that series of patients from 22 percent (in 1968) to about 50 percent. The longest surviving cardiac transplant patient has lived over five years following operation. The majority of patients alive at three months following transplantation have great improvement in symptoms. Although the initial long-term survival figures have been disappointing, they compare not unfavorably with those achieved in renal transplantation at a corresponding stage of its development. However, the difficulty in obtaining suitable donor hearts and the problems with rejection of transplanted tissues by the body may preclude wide clinical application of heart transplantation. Such difficulties have stimulated those researchers committed to an alternate solution, the development of an artificial heart.

Assisted Circulation and the Artificial Heart

Considerable effort has been directed toward the development of devices which will temporarily assist the circulation for days or weeks during periods of unusual stress such as severe heart failure, or following a serious heart attack (see Chapter 7). Such external devices also might be used to keep a patient alive while preparing for conventional heart surgery or for heart transplantation. They have sometimes been helpful postoperatively, in helping patients to survive after a difficult cardiac operation. Relatively short-term assistance to the heart for hours and days has now been accomplished in a number of cardiac centers, and a variety of new approaches are under development. One such procedure currently employed to support patients having shock or low blood pressure, such as may follow a heart attack, is "balloon counterpulsation." This procedure can prove lifesaving by temporarily relieving the load on the heart and elevating the patient's blood pressure. It works by a simple but ingenious principle: A balloon at the end of a plastic tube or catheter is inserted through an artery in the leg and positioned under the fluoroscope to lie in the aorta. After each heartbeat, the balloon is inflated transiently during ventricular relaxation for a few seconds thereby raising the pressure in the aorta and improving blood flow into the coronary arteries of the heart and other vessels leading from the aorta. Subsequently, the balloon is rapidly deflated during the heart's pumping cycle, allowing the left ventricle to eject easily against a relatively low pressure. This cycle is repeated with each heartbeat. It may be expected that the next few years will see many advances and improvements in this and other methods for assisting the circulation by externally connected devices.

The problem of developing an artificial heart that would be completely implanted within the body has been fraught with difficulty, although in animals it has now been possible to implant artificial hearts inside the chest that have supported the circulation for some weeks. One complexity in the problem is made evident by referring to the circulation through the normal heart (Figure 1-1). The heart is two pumps—one supplying venous blood to the lungs, the other supplying oxygenated blood to the aorta, and these pumps must work together. Nevertheless, several types of dual pumps which have artificial pumping chambers and valves have been developed for this purpose. Methods for connecting the pump to the veins and the arteries leading from the heart also have been devised. However, at least two major problem areas remain: Artificial materials that are compatible with blood for long periods of time (surfaces that do not clot or destroy blood cells) are needed, and sources of power to reliably activate the pumping chambers over long periods of time are required. However, it is possible that in the not too distant future total heart replacement, either by an implanted artificial device or by transplantation, will become available for patients whose hearts are damaged beyond the possibility of adequate drug therapy or ordinary surgical repair.

REFERENCES

General

Cardiovascular Surgery, U.S. Department of Health, Education and Welfare, Public Health Service, Bethesda, Maryland.

Johnson, S. L., *The History of Cardiac Surgery 1894–1955*, The Johns Hopkins Press, Baltimore, 1970.

Richardson, R. G., *The Scalpel and the Heart*, Charles Scribner and Sons, New York, 1970.

Willius, F. A., and Keys, T. E., *Cardiac Classics*, C. V. Mosby, St. Louis, Mo., 1941.

Scientific Works

Clark, D. A., Stinson, E. B., Griepp, R. B., Schroeder, J. S., Shumway, N. E., Harrison, D. C., "Cardiac Transplantation in Man. VI. Prognosis of Patients Selected for Cardiac Transplantation," *Annals of Internal Medicine*, **75**:14, 1971.

Kawai, J., Volder, J., Donovan, F. M., Kolff, W. J., "Long term effects of the artificial heart," *Annals of Surgery*, **179**:362–371, 1974.

Kouchoukos, N. T., and Kirklin, J. W., "Coronary Bypass Operations for Ischemic Heart Disease," *Modern Concepts of Cardiovascular Disease*, **41**:47, 1972.

Nora, J. J., Cooley, D. A., Fernback, D. J., et al., "Rejection of the Transplanted Human Heart, Indexes of Recognition and Problems and Prevention," *New England Journal of Medicine*, **280**:1079, 1969.

Pluth, J. R., and McGoon, D. C., "Current Status of Heart Valve Replacement," *Modern Concepts of Cardiovascular Disease*, **43**:65, 1974.

Glossary

Acetylcholine   A compound released from the endings of nerves which supply the heart. It causes the heart rate to slow.

Actin and myosin   Types of protein strands or filaments within the heart muscle which interact chemically during muscle contraction.

Adams-Stokes attack   Transient loss of consciousness or seizure due to an abnormal heart rhythm, usually complete heart block.

Adrenaline   A hormone released into the bloodstream directly from the adrenal glands during stress which stimulates the heart, speeding the heart rate, increasing the force of the heartbeat, and raising the blood pressure.

Aldosterone   A hormone normally secreted by the adrenal gland, which causes retention of sodium (salt) and loss of potassium in the body.

Aneurysm   An abnormal outpouching or enlargement of the wall of an artery. In a "dissecting aneurysm" of the aorta, a break in the lining allows blood to penetrate into the layers of the aortic wall.

Angina pectoris   Chest pain in patients with coronary heart disease due to inadequate oxygen supply to contracting cardiac muscle. Usually it comes on during exertion.

Angiocardiography X-ray pictures of the heart exposed in rapid sequence as liquid, which is opaque to the x-rays, mixes with the blood. This allows visualization of the heart chambers.

Antibody A serum protein produced by the body tissue in response to a foreign protein stimulus.

Anticoagulants Medications used for thinning the blood (making it less likely to clot).

Antigen A protein substance, foreign to the bloodstream, which stimulates the formation of a specific antibody.

Aorta The single large vessel which arises directly from the left-sided pumping chamber and gives branches to all the organs of the body, supplying them with oxygenated (red) blood.

Aortic regurgitation Leakage or insufficiency of the aortic valve.

Aortic stenosis Narrowing of the aortic valve.

Aortic valve A three-leaflet valve which is normally closed during left-ventricular relaxation and open during contraction of the left ventricle to allow the ejection of blood into the aorta.

Arrhythmia A rhythm disorder of the heart characterized by a changing interval between several heart beats, interference with the passage of an electrical impulse through the conduction system or a heart rate faster or slower than the normal resting range of 60 to 100 beats per minute.

Arteriography Injection of x-ray contrast liquid into an artery by means of a catheter so that the artery can be visualized on the x-ray.

Arteriosclerosis "Hardening" of the arteries, often associated with age, but also usually accompanied by atherosclerosis.

Atherogenesis The formation of yellow plaques containing cholesterol and fats on the inner wall of the arteries.

Atherosclerosis A progressive build up of fatty materials within the walls of the arterial blood vessels leading to narrowing or actual blockage of the channel within the involved vessel.

Atomic pacemaker (See Electrical pacemaker.) Utilizes an atomic energy source rather than a pacemaker battery pack.

Atrial fibrillation A heart rhythm in which there are rapid, ineffective irregular atrial contractions at a rate of 400 to 600 per minute and a slower rate response of the ventricles. The pumping of the ventricles is effective, however, and long survival is usual with this disorder.

Atrial septal defect   A hole between the two receiving chambers (atria) of the heart.

Atrial tachycardia   An abnormal rapid regular heart rhythm originating in the atria, outside the sinus node (the heart's normal pacemaker).

Atrioventricular node   A small collection of specialized conducting tissue where the electrical impulse is delayed for less than one-thousandth of a second. It lies between the receiving and pumping chambers.

Atrium   Receiving chamber of the heart. The right atrium receives venous blood from the body, the left atrium, oxygenated blood from the lungs.

Atropine   A medication, used to treat gastrointestinal spasm and certain eye troubles, which increases the heart rate. It counteracts the effects of acetylcholine.

Automaticity   The ability of a heart cell to generate spontaneously an electrical impulse.

Autonomic nervous system   A system of nerve cells whose activities are beyond voluntary control. It includes the sympathetic and parasympathetic nervous systems.

Bacterial endocarditis   Infection on a normal or diseased heart valve causing tissue destruction and abnormal valve function.

Balloon counterpulsation   A balloon in the aorta electronically triggered to inflate during the rest phase of the cardiac cycle and to deflate during the contraction phase. This device, which helps push blood through the coronary arteries, is effective for temporary support of the circulation.

Beta-blocking drugs   Drugs which block the increases in heart rate and strength of heart muscle contraction resulting from sympathetic nervous system stimulation or epinephrine release from the adrenal glands.

Blalock-Taussig operation   An operation designed to increase the amount of blood which passes through the lungs by attaching the end of one of the arm arteries to the pulmonary artery. Used to treat cyanotic children (blue babies).

Blood pressure   The pressure of the blood contained within the arteries. It is maintained by the contraction of the left ventricle and the resistance of the small arteries.

Blood vessel   A tube (artery, capillary, or vein) which transports the blood.

Bradycardia   A heart rate less than sixty beats per minute.

Bruit   A sound in the heart or a blood vessel heard with the stethoscope.

Calcium   The element responsible for activating the contraction process in heart muscle. It is also sometimes deposited in diseased blood vessels and heart valves.

Capillary   A tiny blood vessel, invisible to the naked eye, which connects arteries to veins within the tissues. Its thin wall allows exchange of nutriments and gases.

Cardiac   Pertaining to the heart.

Cardiac arrest   Absence of an effective heartbeat. Caused by complete cessation of electrical activity, or ventricular fibrillation. Frequently caused by a heart attack.

Cardiac output   The amount of blood ejected by the heart during each minute.

Cardiologist   A physician internist specializing in diseases of the heart and blood vessels.

Carotid sinus stimulation   The application of transient pressure over the carotid artery in the neck to terminate atrial tachycardias.

Catheter   A small hollow plastic tube that is passed within the arteries or veins to reach the heart. It is used to measure pressures inside the heart and to inject liquid used for x-ray studies.

Cell membrane   A thin layer of tissue which serves as the enveloping capsule of the cell.

Chelating agents   Chemical substances which have been purported, incorrectly, to remove calcium and cholesterol from arteries affected with atherosclerosis.

Cholesterol   A major fatty substance found in the bloodstream and in tissue which is produced by the liver and is present in the diet. Elevated blood cholesterol levels are associated with an increased risk of coronary heart disease.

Cineangiography   (See Angiocardiography.) High-speed motion pictures for x-ray visualization of the heart and blood vessels after injection of contrast liquid.

Claudication   Leg pains during exercise resulting from atherosclerosis which partially blocks the arteries to the leg.

Clofibrate   A drug which probably interferes with cholesterol production by the liver.

Closed-heart surgery   Cardiac operations during which the heart beats normally and supports the circulation.

Coarctation of the aorta   An area of narrowing in the aorta, a considerable distance away from the heart, present at birth.

Collateral blood vessels   Blood vessels which develop around a blocked artery and are able to compensate in part for the loss of blood supply.

Commissurotomy A heart operation in which the fused leaflets of a scarred valve are opened.

Common (His) bundle A specialized electrical conduction pathway in the heart which divides into a slim right bundle branch and a larger left bundle branch.

Conduction system A system of specialized heart tissue which permits the rapid transmission of electrical impulses from the sinus node to the muscle of the right and left ventricles.

Congenital Inborn.

Congestive heart failure The build-up of fluid in the tissues of the legs and the lungs of patients with reduced heart function.

Constrictive pericarditis Scarring of the sac around the heart (pericardium) leading to poor heart function.

Contrast medium (liquid) A substance that is not penetrated by x-rays that is injected into the blood to visualize the heart and arteries.

Coronary (See Coronary artery.) A term sometimes used to describe a heart attack, or myocardial infarction.

Coronary arteries Blood vessels which originate from the aorta and carry oxygenated blood to nourish the contracting heart muscle.

Coronary arteriography The injection of liquid through a catheter directly into the left and right coronary arteries during the exposure of x-ray pictures in rapid sequence to define the anatomy of the coronary arteries.

Coronary occlusion Obstruction of a coronary artery by atherosclerosis, sometimes with blood clot formation. A heart attack often results.

Coronary prone An individual with several risk factors for the early development of heart disease.

Coumadin A class of blood-thinning medications which interfere with clotting factors made by the liver, and delay blood clotting.

Countershock The use of direct current discharge to revert rapid heart rhythm to normal rhythm.

Cyanosis Blueness of the skin due to low oxygen content of the blood in the arteries.

Defibrillation Electric shock applied to terminate atrial or ventricular fibrillation and to restore a normal heartbeat.

Depolarization A loss in the resting electrical charge of heart muscle cells upon the arrival of an electrical impulse initiated by specialized cells. Depolarization initiates contraction.

Diabetes mellitus A metabolic disorder in which the ability to break down carbohydrates is lost due to insufficient insulin production by the pancreas.

Diastole The rest phase of the heart cycle in which the pumping chambers fill.

Diastolic blood pressure The lowest blood pressure recorded with each heart cycle. Occurs during the heart's relaxation phase.

Digitalis A heart medication which markedly strengthens the beat of the failing heart and is effective in slowing excessively rapid heart action in certain heart rhythm disorders.

Disc valve An artificial valve prosthesis which has either a tilting disc or a disc moving within a small cage.

Diuretics Medications which increase the amount of urine excretion.

Dropsy A term formerly used to denote generalized swelling of the body.

Ectopic beat A heartbeat that arises in any site outside the normal sinus pacemaker.

Edema An excessive accumulation of fluid in the body tissues.

Electrical impulse An electrical signal initiated in pacemaker cells and transmitted through the cardiac conduction system to initiate heart muscle contraction.

Electrical pacemaker An electrode-tipped tube positioned in the right ventricle which uses a battery pack to initiate the heart's electrical impulse.

Electrical potential The difference in electrical charge between the inside and the outside of the cell membrane.

Electrocardiogram A graphic representation of the electrical currents which initiate each heart cycle, as recorded from the surface of the body.

Electron microscope A microscope with many times the magnification of an ordinary microscope which uses electrons rather than light to delineate the object.

Electrophoresis The movement of particles in an electric field toward the positive or negative electric pole.

Embolus A blood clot which dislodges from its site of formation and is carried in the bloodstream to lodge in the lungs (pulmonary embolus), or to other organs of the body when it arises in the left side of the heart.

Emphysema Overinflation of the lungs which usually results from chronic disease of the air passages.

Endocardium   The inner layer of tissue which separates heart muscle from blood.

Enzyme   A compound contained in a cell which is capable of accelerating a chemical reaction within the body. Its release from the cell into the bloodstream is often an indication of cell damage.

Epicardium   The thin outer layer of tissue which covers the heart muscle.

Epinephrine   One of the hormones secreted by the adrenal gland (see Adrenaline).

Essential hypertension   An elevated arterial blood pressure for which no specific cause is apparent.

Exercise electrocardiogram   An electrocardiogram recorded continuously during progressive exercise (usually on a treadmill). Used to detect abnormalities in the recovery phase of the electrocardiogram during stress in patients with coronary artery disease.

External cardiac massage   Maintenance of the circulation by regular external compression of the chest.

Fabric-covered prosthesis   An artificial valve with a thin layer of cloth covering the metal base and the metal struts.

Fibrillation   Rapid, disorganized beating of either the atria (receiving chambers) or ventricles (pumping chambers). (See Atrial and ventricular fibrillation.)

Filaments   Small protein strands within each muscle cell which slide over one another during contraction.

Functional murmur   A soft murmur often heard in the normal heart, particularly in children and young adults, due simply to the rapid circulation of blood across normal heart valves.

Gallop   A thudding sound heard in the abnormal heart which often signifies disease of the heart muscle.

Guanethidine   A potent drug used in the treatment of patients with hypertension which prevents the release of norepinephrine from the nerve terminals.

Heart attack   Death of heart muscle due to a coronary occlusion or insufficient coronary blood flow to meet the oxygen needs of the muscle. It is usually associated with severe, prolonged chest pain, and there may be sudden and serious rhythm disorders.

Heart block   Interference with the passage of the electrical impulse through the heart's conduction system.

Heart failure   Inability of the heart to eject a sufficient amount of blood per minute to satisfy the demands of the body tissues. Often it is associated with a high pressure in the veins draining the lungs and body tissues.

Heart-lung machine   An artificial circulatory support device used during open heart surgery.

Heart transplantation   The implantation of a donor's heart into the chest of a recipient to replace a severely diseased heart.

Hemoglobin   An iron-containing protein substance contained in the blood cells which binds gases readily, particularly oxygen.

Heterograft valve   A valve prosthesis which uses a tissue valve obtained from animal species other than man, such as swine.

His bundle   (See Common bundle.)

Homograft valve   A valve prosthesis which uses a normal human valve obtained at the time of an autopsy performed under sterile conditions.

Hormone   A chemical substance formed in one organ or part of the body and carried in the blood to another organ or tissue, which it stimulates to functional activity.

Hydralazine   A drug which reduces the blood pressure by decreasing the resistance to blood flow in the small arteries.

Hyperlipidemia   Elevation of certain fats (cholesterol and/or triglycerides) above their normal concentrations in the blood.

Hypertension   A state of abnormally elevated blood pressure, frequently associated with structural and functional abnormalities of many organs including the blood vessels, heart, and kidneys.

Hypertrophy   Increase in the amount of heart muscle tissue associated with chronic enlargement of the heart usually due to long standing valvular heart disease or high blood pressure.

Immunity   Protection against a particular disease or foreign substance, as a result of antibody formation.

Immunosuppressive drugs   Medications used to prevent antibody formation by the body in response to a foreign tissue. Used to prevent cardiac rejection in patients undergoing heart transplantation.

Internal mammary artery implantation   The insertion of a chest wall artery (the internal mammary artery) directly into cardiac muscle to increase its nutrient blood supply.

Ion   An element or group of molecules which carry a charge of electricity.

Isoproterenol   A medication which increases the heart rate and force of heart contraction.

Left atrium   A thin-walled muscular heart chamber situated behind the left ventricle which receives oxygenated (red) blood from the lungs.

Left ventricle   A thick-walled muscular chamber responsible for pumping oxygenated blood into the aorta and general circulation.

Lidocaine   Medication given by venous injection to prevent arrhythmias in patients with a recent heart attack.

Lipids   Fatty substances circulating in the blood, including triglycerides and cholesterol.

Lipoproteins   Circulating proteins to which the blood lipids are attached.

Membrane oxygenator   A device in which blood is passed within a series of thin plastic films, which allows exchange of oxygen and carbon dioxide without direct contact between gas and blood.

Methyldopa   A drug, frequently used in the treatment of hypertension, which displaces norepinephrine from the nerve terminals.

Mitral commissurotomy   A closed heart operation for the relief of mitral valve narrowing in which the surgeon separates the adherent leaflets with his finger or a knife.

Mitral regurgitation   Insufficiency or leakage of the mitral valve.

Mitral stenosis   Narrowing of the mitral valve.

Mitral valve   The two leaflet valve between the left atrium and ventricle which is normally closed during left-ventricular contraction and open during left-ventricular filling.

Murmur   A vibration within the heart heard through the stethoscope. Usually produced by the rushing of blood across an abnormal heart valve.

Myocardial disease   Disease primarily affecting the muscle of the heart.

Myocardial infarction   The medical term usually employed to indicate death of heart muscle (heart attack).

Myocarditis   An infectious disease resulting in inflammatory reaction in heart muscle.

Myocardium   Heart muscle.

Nitroglycerin   A medication used in the treatment of angina pectoris which dilates the coronary arteries and lowers the oxygen demands on the heart by reducing the blood pressure.

Norepinephrine   A substance released from nerve fibers which supply the heart. It increases the heart rate and causes the heart muscle to contract more forcefully.

Open-heart surgery   Heart operations in which the heart is opened while it is empty of blood. A heart-lung machine is used to support the circulation.

Oxygen consumption   The uptake of oxygen from the arterial blood by the body tissue.

Oxygenated blood Blood which has received oxygen while passing through the lungs.

Oxygenator The portion of a heart-lung machine which provides a large surface area for exchange of oxygen and carbon dioxide.

P wave A small deflection of the surface electrocardiogram which represents atrial depolarization.

Pacemaker The site from which an electrical impulse driving the heart originates. The normal heart pacemaker is the sinus node.

Palpitation An unpleasant sensation of the heartbeat, or of a skipped heartbeat.

Papillary muscles Small muscles attached to the heart walls within the right and left ventricles which help to support the tricuspid and mitral valves.

Paroxysmal tachycardia Rapid heart action that begins and ends suddenly.

Parasympathetic nervous system That portion of the autonomic nervous system which releases acetylcholine at its nerve terminals, which decreases the heart rate.

Patent ductus arteriosus A connection between the aorta and pulmonary artery which normally closes shortly after birth.

Pericardium The thin membrane which envelopes the heart like a sack, holding it in position within the chest.

Pericarditis Inflammation of the pericardium.

Permeability That property of a membrane which allows the passage of liquids into and out of the cell.

Pheochromocytoma A type of tumor of the adrenal gland which produces epinephrine and norepinephrine in excess.

Phlebitis Inflammation of the veins, which may result in clot formation ("thrombophlebitis").

Phonocardiogram The graphic representation of the heart sounds and heart murmurs using a small microphone applied to the skin over the heart. The sounds are amplified and recorded on moving paper.

Pneumatic cuff The inflatable rubber bag which is placed around the arm for the measurement of blood pressure.

Poppet A silicone or metallic ball which moves between the metal base and the struts of the cage in a heart valve prosthesis.

Premature beat An extra beat that occurs earlier than the next expected normal heartbeat.

Pressure gradient A difference in pressure measured across a narrowed heart valve.

Procainamide   A medication used for the treatment of abnormal cardiac rhythms, particularly ventricular arrhythmias.

Propranolol   A medication which blocks the effects of epinephrine and stimulation of the sympathetic nervous system on heart rate and the force of heart contraction. It is used in the treatment of angina pectoris and certain abnormal heart rhythms.

Prosthesis   A device used to replace a natural organ or structure (such as a heart valve).

Pulmonary artery   A large blood vessel which carries venous blood from the right ventricle to the lungs.

Pulmonary circulation   The network of vessels which carry blood from the right ventricle through the pulmonary artery to the lungs and back through the pulmonary veins to the left atrium (as distinct from the systemic circulation).

Pulmonary edema   Marked accumulation of fluid in the air sacs of the lungs, usually resulting from disease of the left side of the heart.

Pulmonary vein   A blood vessel which transports oxygenated blood from the lungs to the left atrium.

Pulmonic valve   A three-leaflet valve which is normally closed during right-ventricular relaxation and open during right-ventricular contraction to allow ejection of blood into the pulmonary artery.

Pulse   The rhythmical expansion of an artery produced by the increased volume of blood flowing into the vessel with each contraction of the heart.

Purkinje cells   Specialized muscle cells in the pumping chambers of the heart concerned primarily with the conduction of the electrical impulses.

QRS complex   A large signal on the surface electrocardiogram which represents depolarization of the ventricles.

Quinidine   A drug derived from the cinchona bark which is used in the treatment of abnormal heart rhythms.

Renin   A protein material released from the kidney into the bloodstream which is essential for the production of angiotensin, a substance which increases blood pressure by causing constriction of the small arteries and also stimulates aldosterone secretion.

Repolarization   The recovery of the initial resting electrical charge of heart muscle cells following electrical depolarization.

Reserpine   A drug used for the treatment of hypertension which decreases the amount of norepinephrine stored in the sympathetic nerve endings which supply the heart and the blood vessels.

Revascularization operations   Surgical procedures used to increase the blood supply to heart muscle.

Rheumatic fever   An allergic reaction to streptococcal bacteria resulting in damage to certain body tissues including the heart valves.

Rheumatic heart disease   Disease of one or more heart valves due to scarring as a consequence of acute rheumatic fever.

Right atrium   A thin-walled muscular heart chamber situated behind the right ventricle which receives (blue) venous blood from the large veins which drain the body.

Right ventricle   A muscular heart chamber which pumps unoxygenated venous blood to the lungs through the pulmonary arteries.

Roller pumps   A type of mechanical pump used in heart-lung machines in which plastic or rubber tubing is gently milked by rotating arms fitted with rollers.

Rubella   German measles. This infection during the first three months of pregnancy is associated with an increased incidence of congenital heart disease in the newborn infant.

St. Vitus' Dance   Involuntary movements of the body which result from involvement of the brain during acute rheumatic fever.

Saphenous vein bypass grafting   A surgical procedure in which the saphenous vein, a superficial vein of the leg, is removed and connected from the aorta to the diseased coronary vessel beyond the site of narrowing of the coronary artery.

Scarlet fever   A skin rash associated with a streptococcal infection.

Secondary hypertension   An elevated blood pressure associated with a specific disorder such as kidney disease.

Septum   Muscular partition or wall inside the heart. The atrial septum divides the two receiving chambers, and the ventricular septum the two pumping chambers of the heart.

Shunt   Mixing of blood between two of the heart's chambers or vessels resulting from an abnormal hole in the wall (septum) between the chambers or a connection between the vessels.

"Shunting" procedures   Operative techniques (such as Blalock-Taussig operation) used in heart surgery for diverting blood low in oxygen through the lungs.

Sinus node   The normal electrical pacemaker of the heart located in the right atrium.

Spironolactone   A drug used in the treatment of high blood pressure which increases salt and water excretion by the kidneys due to its inhibitor effect on aldosterone secretion from the adrenal gland.

Starling's law of the heart   The amount of blood pumped out by the heart with each beat is determined by the amount of blood which fills it prior to the contraction.

Stenosis Narrowing of a heart valve.

Stroke Damage to the brain caused by occlusion of an artery and loss of blood supply to brain tissue (by atherosclerosis or clot), or damage caused by sudden bleeding into or around the brain.

Sulfadiazine An antibiotic used in the treatment and prevention of streptococcal throat infections.

Sympathetic nervous system That portion of the autonomic nervous system which contains norepinephrine within the nerve endings, the release of which stimulates the heart muscle to increase its rate of beating and strength of contraction.

Systemic circulation The network of vessels which carry blood through the body: the arteries, capillaries, and veins of the general circulation (as distinct from the pulmonary circulation).

Systole The phase of the heart cycle in which the pumping chambers contract to eject blood.

Systolic blood pressure The maximum blood pressure which occurs with each heart cycle during contraction of the left-sided pumping chamber.

T wave A small deflection on the surface electrocardiogram which represents repolarization of the ventricles.

Tachycardia A rapid heart rhythm, with rate over 100 per minute.

Thrombosis Clot within a blood vessel, which may block it.

Thrombophlebitis Inflammation and clot formation within the veins of the body.

Tricuspid valve The three leaflet valve between the right atrium and ventricle which is normally closed during right ventricular contraction and open during right ventricular filling.

Vectorcardiogram A three-dimensional electrocardiogram.

Vena cava Large veins which connect directly to the heart and drain blood from the upper and lower parts of the body.

Venous blood Blood returning from the veins of the body which has not yet passed through the lungs to receive additional oxygen.

Ventricle Pumping chamber of the heart. The right ventricle pumps venous blood to the lungs, the left ventricle, oxygenated blood to the body.

Ventricular fibrillation A very rapid chaotic ventricular rhythm associated with completely ineffective ventricular contractions which rapidly results in death if not promptly treated.

Ventricular septal defect   A hole in the septum between the left and right sided pumping chambers (ventricles) of the heart.

Ventricular tachycardia   A dangerous, abnormal heart rhythm originating in the ventricle with a rapid heart rate between 120 and 180 beats per minute.

Vitamin E   A deficiency of this vitamin has been associated with heart disease in experimental animals but not in human beings. This vitamin is of no proven efficacy in the treatment or prevention of cardiac disease in man.

Wolff-Parkinson-White syndrome   A syndrome associated with an abnormal conduction pathway between the atria and the ventricles which allows the electrical impulses to bypass the atrioventricular node. Recurrent paroxysmal atrial tachycardia often occurs with this syndrome.

INDEX

Acetycholine, 21–23
Actin, 17
Adams-Stokes attacks, 74
Adrenal glands, 21, 111, 118, 123
Adrenalin:
  in heart failure, 123
  regulating heart beat, 21–23, 79
Age, as a risk factor, 89
Alcohol, effects on heart, 54–55, 79, 122
Aldosterone, hypertension and, 113–114, 117, 118
Amino acids, 2–3, 7, 49
Amphetamines:
  disorders of heart rhythm, 77
  effects on the heart, 60
Anemia, 79
Anesthetic agents, 82
Anesthetic techniques, 145

Aneurysm, aortic, in hypertension, 116
Angina pectoris:
  definition of, 89, 92
  mechanism, 92–94
  treatment for, 103–105, 151–154
Angiocardiography:
  in congenital heart disease, 132–133
  diagnostic technique, 26, 40–42
Angiotensin, 114
Antibiotics and rheumatic fever, 63
Anticoagulants:
  in mitral stenosis, 71
  with prosthetic valves, 149
Antigens, 63, 155
Antihypertensive drugs, 117–119
Aorta:
  anatomy and function, 3, 13, 28, 67
  aneurysm of, 116

Aorta:
  angiography, 42
  assisted circulation, 106
  catheterization of, 38–39
  coronary artery surgery, 104–105
  echocardiogram of, 35
Aortic valve:
  angiocardiography of, 42
  bacterial infection of, 59
  catheterization of, 38–40
  heart murmurs, 27–28
  normal function, 13
  prosthesis (artificial valve), 148–150
  regurgitation (insufficiency), 67, 123
  rheumatic fever and, 63–64
  stenosis of, 28, 67–68, 123
  surgical replacement of, 148–150
Arrhythmias:
  atrial fibrillation, 66–67, 70–71, 80
  atrial premature beats, 76
  atrial tachycardia, 79–80
  definition, 74
  extra beats, 76–78
  heart block, 83–85
  sinus bradycardia, 83
  sinus tachycardia, 78–79
  treatment, 85–87
  ventricular fibrillation, 81–82, 96,
    106
  ventricular premature beats, 76–77
  ventricular tachycardia, 81–82
Arteries:
  anatomy and function, 1–7, 20–23
  atherosclerosis of, 99, 116
  cardiac catheterization of, 35–39
  constriction of, 113
  high blood pressure, 115–116
  pulse wave form of, 34
Arteriosclerosis (see Atherosclerosis)
Artificial heart, 156–158
Artificial heart valve (prosthesis), 69–
    70, 127, 147–150
Artificial respiration, 106
Artificial support systems, 106, 146–
    147
Assisted circulation, 106, 156–157

Atherogenic diet, 46
Atherosclerosis:
  age, 91
  cholesterol, 99–103
  cigarette smoking, 91
  coronary arteries, 17, 26, 41, 45, 88,
    91
  diabetes, 91
  diet, 46–47, 91, 130
  heart failure in, 129
  high blood pressure in, 91, 115–116,
    119
  lipids, 90–91
  lipoproteins, 99–103
  triglycerides, 99–103
Athletes, 55–56
Atomic pacemaker, 87
Atrial contractions, 80
Atrial fibrillation, 66, 70–71, 80
Atrial impulses, 80
Artrial muscle, 76
Atrial premature beats, 76–78
Atrial septal defect, 139, 142, 151
Atrial tachycardia, 79–80
Atrioventricular (AV) node:
  anatomy and function, 15, 75–76
  digitalis, 81
  electrical impuse, 75–76
  electrocardiogram, 30
  heart block, 83–85
Atrium:
  in atrial fibrillation, 80
  conduction system of, 15, 29, 74
  electrocardiogram of, 29
  in heart transplantation, 155
  left, 3, 9–10, 38–40, 64–66, 70, 139,
    145
  pacemaker site in, 15, 74
  right, 3, 8, 15, 139
Atromid, 102
Atropine, 23, 79, 87

Bacterial endocarditis, 70
Bacterial infection:
  of heart muscle, 121–122

Bacterial infection:
  of heart valves, 14–15, 59
  of pericardium, 29, 122
  rheumatic fever, 63
Balloon counterpulsation, 106–107, 157
Behavior patterns, 56–57
Beta-adrenergic blocking agents:
  in angina pectoris, 103–104
  in high blood pressure, 117, 118
Blalock-Taussig operation, 140–141
Blood clots, 10, 67, 70–71, 140, 149
Blood glucose, 98
Blood lipids, 26, 46, 90, 98–103
Blood pressure, 3–7, 22–23, 56, 91, 97, 109–111
Blood thinning agents, 71, 149
Blood transfusion, 145
"Blue baby" operations, 134, 140–141
Bradycardia, 83–85
Brain:
  atherosclerosis of, 89
  high blood pressure and, 116
  regulating heart beat, 21–22
Bruit, 28
Bypass graft surgery, 105, 127, 152

Caged ball valve prosthesis, 148–149
Calcium:
  in atherosclerosis, 102
  chelating agents, 102
  digitalis and, 129
  heart contraction and, 17–20, 126
Capillaries:
  anatomy and function, 1–2, 7, 9–10
  coronary circulation, 17
  pulmonary circulation, 9, 37
Carbohydrates, 46–48, 98, 101
Cardiac arrest, 82, 95, 105
Cardiac catheterization, 35–40, 42, 65, 133, 138, 142, 152
Cardiac neurosis, 42
Cardiac output, 118
Cardiac rehabilitation centers, 51
Cardiac rhythm abnormalities, 73

Cardiologist, 2
Cardioversion, 82
Carotid artery, 80
Carotid sinus stimulation, 80
Catheter, 35–39, 85, 106
Cell membrane, 15
Central nervous system, 21
Chelating agents, 102
Cholesterol:
  blood levels, 26, 46–47, 56, 89–91, 98–100
  deposits, 89, 103
Cholestyramine, 102
Cigarette smoking, 45, 52–53, 59, 91, 98
Cineangiocardiography, 40, 134
Circulation:
  assisted, 106
  coronary, 17
  cross, 145
  pulmonary, 8–10
  systemic, 3–10
Claudication, 89
Clofibrate, 102
Closed heart surgery, 145
Coarctation of the aorta, 111, 117, 134–135
Collateral blood vessels, 97
Common bundle, 75
Complete heart block, 73, 84–86
Conducting fibers, 15
Conduction system:
  anatomy and function, 12, 15
  electrocardiogram and, 29–30
  in heart attack, 32–33, 105
  in heart block, 60, 83
  in myocardial disease, 122
Congenital heart disease (see Inborn heart defects)
Continuous electrocardiographic monitoring, 74, 78, 105
Contraction, 10, 13, 21, 28, 32, 67
Coronary arteries:
  anatomy and function, 17
  arteriography (angiography) of, 40–42, 105, 149

Coronary artery disease:
  arrhythmias in, 105–106
  atrial fibrillation in, 80–81
  blood lipids in, 98–103
  bypass operation for, 42, 105, 152–153
  cause, 88–90
  electrocardiogram in, 32
  exercise electrocardiogram in, 33
  heart attack, 95–97, 105–106
  heart failure in, 123
  heart pain, 92–94
  incidence of, 88, 90
  risk factors for, 46, 91–92
  valve disease and, 65
Coronary blood flow, 152
Coronary care units, 74, 105–106
"Coronary prone" individuals, 56, 97–98
Coronary surgery, 151–154
Coumadin, 71
Countershock, 74, 81–82
Cross circulation, 145
Cyanosis, 132, 134, 140–141

Defibrillation, 82, 105
Depolarization, 15, 29, 30, 82
Dexedrine, 60
Diabetes mellitus, 46–47, 91, 130
Diagnostic studies, 25
Diastole, 148
Diastolic blood pressure, 6, 109–111, 115, 117, 119
Diet:
  atherosclerosis, 47, 90
  fad, 48
  familial hypercholesterolemia, 101
  gelatin, 48
  high protein-high water, 48
  hypoglycemic, 48
  low salt, 49
  skim milk and bananas, 48
  weight reducing, 47–48
Digitalis:
  in atrial fibrillation, 70–71, 80

Digitalis:
  in atrial tachycardia, 79
  excess of, 76
  in heart failure, 127–129
  in valvular heart disease, 69–70
Disc valve, 148
Diuretic agents:
  in heart failure, 127, 129
  in high blood pressure, 117, 118
  in valvular heart disease, 70
Drugs:
  abuse of, 59–60
  antihypertensive agents, 117–119
  congenital heart disease, 58

Echocardiogram, 26, 34–35
Edema, 66, 125
Electrical countershock, 81
Electrical failure, 122
Electrical impulses, 15, 29–30, 74, 78, 124, 128
Electrical instability, 105
Electrical pacemaker, 15, 22, 85–87, 122
Electrical system, 73
Electrocardiogram:
  in coronary artery disease, 32
  exercise, 33
  in heart block, 83
  normal tracing, 15–16, 29–30
  premature beats, 76–77
  in ventricular enlargement, 32
  in Wolff-Parkinson-White syndrome, 80
Electrode, 15, 29–30, 32, 85
Electronic evaluation, 86
Electronic monitoring system, 74
Electronic pacemaker, 74, 85–87
Electronic transducer, 39
Electrophoresis, 99
Embolus, 10, 67, 71
Emotional stress, 21, 56–57, 78
Emphysema, 125
Epicardial abrasion, 151
Epicardium, 151

Escape rhythm, 75
Exercise:
   coronary artery disease, 50–52
   electrocardiographic testing, 33
   rehabilitation, 51–52
External cardiac massage, 106
Extra beats, 59, 76–78

Fabric-covered artificial valves, 149
Familial:
   coronary artery disease, 90
   high blood pressure, 113
   hypercholesterolemia, 47, 99, 101
   hyperlipidemia, 47, 99, 100
   hypertriglyceridemia, 100, 101
Fat:
   artery deposits, 89, 92, 95
   blood levels, 89, 101–102
Fibrillation:
   atrial, 66, 70–71, 80
   ventricular, 81–82, 96, 106
Filaments, 17, 24, 125–126
Fluoroscope, 157
Foreign proteins, 63
Functional murmurs, 27

Gallop sounds, 26
Gastrointestinal antispasmodics, 79
German measles (see Rubella)
Glomerulonephritis, 63, 64
Grafts:
   coronary artery bypass, 42, 152
   tissue valves, 149–150
Guanethidine, 118

Hardening of the arteries (see Atherosclerosis)
Heart attack:
   arrhythmias, 81, 82, 84, 105
   coronary arteries, 17
   electrocardiogram, 32–33
   heart block, 83–85, 104–105
   heart failure, 23–24

Heart attack:
   lidocaine, 78, 81
   mechanism, 95–97
   symptoms, 95–97
   treatment, 105–107
   ventricular tachycardia, 81
Heart block:
   atropine, 87
   causes, 83–85
   definition, 73–74, 83
   in heart attack, 84, 105
   in heart failure, 122–123
   pacemaker, 85–87
   treatment of, 85–87
Heart chambers:
   general, 3, 5–10, 13–14, 23, 39–40
   left atrium, 3, 9, 37–38, 40, 54, 65,
     67, 70, 139, 142, 145
   left ventricle, 3–4, 9–10, 28, 32, 37–
     38, 40, 54, 65, 67–69, 116, 138–
     140, 153, 157
   right atrium, 35, 139, 142
   right ventricle, 3, 9, 35, 69, 125, 137,
     139–142
Heart failure:
   aldosterone, 113–114
   causes, 121–124
   digitalis, 126–129
   effects, 124–126
   in heart attack, 23–24
   in high blood pressure, 116
   prevention of, 129–130
   sinus tachycardia, 78–79
   treatment of, 127–129
   valvular heart disease, 64–65
Heart-lung bypass, 145
Heart-lung machine, 139–141, 146–
   147, 155
Heart murmurs:
   in aortic regurgitation, 27, 64
   in aortic stenosis, 28, 64
   in congenital heart disease, 138
   definition of, 27
   functional, 27
   location of, 28
   in mitral regurgitation, 28, 64

Heart murmurs:
  in mitral stenosis, 28, 65
  timing of, 28
Heart muscle:
  anatomy and function, 17–20
  disease of, 121–122
  in heart attack, 95–97
  in heart failure, 125–126
  in high blood pressure, 116
Heart rhythm, 30, 32, 73–87
Heart sounds, 26–27
Heart surgery:
  artificial heart, 156–158
  assisted circulation, 106–107, 156–
    158
  in congenital heart disease, 150–151
  in coronary heart disease, 151–154
  heart transplanatation, 154–156
  in valve disease, 69–70, 145–150
Heart transplantation, 154–156
Hemoglobin, 7–9, 52
Heroin, 59
Heterografts, 150
High blood pressure:
  atrial fibrillation, 80
  in coarctation of aorta, 111
  complications, 115–116
  coronary risk factor, 90–92
  detection clinics for, 115
  diagnosis, 5–6, 111–115
  diastolic hypertension, 111
  essential hypertension, 111–115
  familial, 113
  heart failure in, 123
  hormones, 113–114
  treatment of, 117–119
High risk individual, 91, 97–99
Homografts, 150
Hormones, 21–23, 113–114
Hydralazine, 117–119
Hypertension (see High blood pres-
    sure)
Hyperthyroidism, 79, 80
Hypertrophy, 123
Hyperventilation, 53

Ileal bypass operation, 103
Immunosuppressive drugs, 155–156
Inborn heart defects:
  angiocardiography in, 40, 133
  aortic stenosis, 135
  atrial septal defect, 134, 139
  Blalock-Taussig operation, 141
  cardiac catheterization, 39, 133
  classification of, 134
  coarctation of the aorta, 134–135
  German measles and, 58, 133
  heart block in, 84–85
  heart failure in, 125
  incidence of, 132
  patent ductus arteriosus, 134, 138
  pulmonic stenosis, 137–138
  surgical treatment of, 137–138,
    150–151
  tetralogy of Fallot, 140–141
  thalidomide and, 59
  transposition of the great arteries,
    141–142
  ventricular septal defect, 134, 139
Incomplete heart block, 83
Inderal, 80, 104, 118
Indirect blood pressure measurement,
    5, 110
Infection:
  of heart muscle, 122
  of heart valves, 14, 59, 69–70
  of pericardium, 29, 122
Internal mammary artery implanta-
    tion, 152
Intracardiac pacemaker, 85–87
Involuntary nervous system:
  atrial tachycardia, 80
  atropine, 87
  in blood pressure regulation, 110,
    113
  drugs, 103–104
  in heart failure, 124
  maneuvers to stimulate, 80
Ions:
  calcium, 18–20, 102, 126
  cell membrane and, 15

Ions:
  digitalis and, 127–129
  potassium, 77, 127
  sodium, 49, 127
Irregular heart rhythm, 74
Isometric exercise, 52
Isoproterenol, 87

Kidneys:
  diseases causing hypertension, 111
  edema and, 125
  glomerulonephritis, 63–64
  in heart failure, 127
  in high blood pressure, 114
  renin release, 114

Leaflets:
  aortic valve, 13, 38, 64–65, 135
  mitral valve, 14, 38, 64, 67, 145–146
  pulmonic valve, 13, 69, 137–138
  synthetic, 148
  tricuspid valve, 13–14, 69
Left atrium:
  anatomy and function, 3, 5, 9
  angiocardiography of, 40
  atrial fibrillation and, 66–67, 70–71
  blood clot in, 67, 70–71
  catheterization of, 38
  in mitral stenosis, 54, 65–67
  and mitral valve surgery, 146
Left bundle branch, 75, 85
Left coronary artery, 17, 152
Left heart catheterization, 38–39
Left ventricle:
  anatomy and function, 3, 5, 9
  angiocardiography of, 40
  in aortic regurgitation, 29, 69
  in aortic stenosis, 28, 67–69, 135
  catheterization of, 38–39
  in coarctation of the aorta, 134–135
  in coronary artery disease, 96, 123
  enlargement of electrocardiogram,
    32–33
  in heart failure, 123–124

Left ventricle:
  in mitral regurgitation, 67
Lidocaine, 78
Lipids:
  atherosclerosis and, 90–91
  blood levels, 26, 46, 91, 98–99
  coronary risk factor, 91, 98–99
  diet and, 47–48
Lungs:
  blood clot in, 10
  circulation, 8–10
  in heart failure, 124–125
  in mitral stenosis, 28, 65–66
  and right heart function, 8–9, 124–
    125

Marihuana, 59
Membrane oxygenator, 147
Methyldopa, 117–118
Mitral regurgitation, 59, 67, 123
Mitral stenosis:
  anticoagulants, 71
  atrial blood clot in, 70–71
  atrial fibrillation in, 66–67, 70
  cardiac catheterization in, 38–39, 65
  cardiac surgery for, 145–147, 150–
    151
  echocardiogram in, 35
  heart examination in, 28, 65
  heart failure in, 65–66, 123
  pressure gradient in, 66–67
  pulmonary edema in, 54, 66
Mitral valve:
  anatomy and function, 14
  cardiac catheterization, 38–39
  echocardiogram of, 35
  heart sounds, 26–27
  infection of, 14, 59
  prosthesis, 69, 148
  regurgitation (see Mitral regurgita-
    tion)
  replacement of, 147–150
  rheumatic fever and, 63–64
  stenosis (see Mitral stenosis)

Mitral valve:
  surgery of, 144–150
Morphine, 83
Murmur (*see* Heart murmur)
Musculoskeletal, 129–130
Myocardial cells, 75–76
Myocardial disease, 122
Myocardial infarction, 95–97
Myocardial revascularization, 152
Myocarditis, 122
Myocardium (*see* Heart muscle)
Myosin, 17

Neosynephrine, 60
Nitroglycerin, 103–104
Node:
  atrioventricular, 15, 29, 30, 75, 79–80, 83
  sinus, 15, 21–22, 29, 75, 79, 83
Noninvasive techniques, 25, 34
Norepinephrine:
  antihypertensive drugs, 117–119
  causing high blood pressure, 113–114
  in heart failure, 124
  regulation of blood pressure, 113
  regulation of heart beat, 22–23

Obesity:
  coronary risk factor, 46, 91
  diets for, 47–49
Open heart surgery, 135, 145–147
Oscilloscope, 34
Oxygenated blood, 3, 9–10, 17, 105, 139–141
Oxygenator, 146–147, 157

P wave, 30, 32, 84
Pacemaker (*see* Electrical pacemaker)
Pacemaker cells, 15, 29, 75
Palpitations, 54, 56, 73, 78
Paroxysmal atrial tachycardia, 79

Patent ductus arteriosus, 138, 145
Penicillin, 64
Pericarditis, 29, 122, 155
Pericardium, 151, 155
Permeability, 15
Phlebitis, 10, 71
Phonocardiogram, 26, 34
Physical examination, 26–29, 65, 115
Pneumatic cuff, 5, 115
Poppet, 148
Potassium, 77, 127
Precordial region, 28
Pregnancy, 57–59
Premature atrial contractions, 76–78
Premature beats, 57, 76–78
Premature ventricular contraction, 53, 76–78, 82
Pressure gradient, 65, 68
Pressure wave, 39
Procaineamide, 78, 80
Progressive exercise training, 50–52, 104
Prophylactic antibiotics, 70
Propranolol, 80, 104, 118–119
Prosthesis, 69, 148
Pulmonary artery, 8, 35, 41, 65, 125, 137–138, 141, 145, 151
Pulmonary circulation, 9
Pulmonary edema, 65
Pulmonary embolus, 10, 71
Pulmonary veins, 9, 54, 65
Pulmonic stenosis, 69, 137–138, 140–141, 151
Pulmonic valve, 13, 26, 69, 137–138, 140–141
Pulse pressure, 5
Pulse rate, 5
Pumping chamber (*see* Ventricles)
Pumping cycle (*see* Systole)
Purkinje cells, 75, 78, 81

Q wave, 32–33
QRS complex, 30, 32–33, 76–77, 84
Quinidine, 78, 80

Rapid heart rate (*see* Tachycardia)
Receiving chamber (*see* Atrium)
Regurgitation:
    aortic, 69, 123
    mitral, 59, 67, 123
    tricuspid, 69
Renin, 114
Repolarization, 32, 33
Reserpine, 117–118
Retrograde catheterization 38
Revascularization, 104, 152
Rheumatic fever, 63–64, 70, 145
Rheumatic heart disease, 14–15, 44,
    54, 64, 69, 76, 122, 149–150
Rhythm disorders (*see* Arrhythmias)
Right atrium:
    anatomy and function, 3, 9
    atrial septal defect, 139
    catheterization of, 35–39
    sinus node, 15, 74
Right bundle, 75, 85
Right coronary artery, 17, 152
Right heart catheterization, 35–36
Right heart failure, 124–125
Right ventricle:
    anatomy and function, 3, 9
    catheterization of, 35–36
    conduction system of, 75
    in heart failure, 125
    pacemaker catheter in, 85–86
    in pulmonic stenosis, 137–138
    rheumatic heart disease, 69
Risk factors (*see* Coronary risk fac-
    tors)
Rubella, 58, 133

St. Vitus' Dance, 63–64
Saphenous vein, 104, 152
Saturated fat, 46, 101
Scarlet fever, 63
Secondary hypertension, 111
Selective coronary angiography, 40–
    42, 152

Septum:
    atrial, 38, 139
    ventricular, 39, 139
Sexual activity, 53–54
Shock, 106
Shunts:
    atrial septal defect, 139, 151
    patent ductus arteriosus, 138, 145
    ventricular septal defect, 39, 139–
    141, 151
Sinus beats, 74–75
Sinus bradycardia, 83
Sinus impulse, 29, 74–75
Sinus node, 15, 21–22, 29, 75–76, 79,
    83–84
Sinus pacemaker, 75–76, 79
Sinus rhythm, 75
Sinus tachycardia, 78–79
Skipped beats, 73, 86
Slow heart rate (*see* Bradycardia)
Spinal cord, 22
Spironolactone, 118
ST segment, 33
Starling's law of the heart, 23–34, 123
Stenosis:
    aortic, 28, 67–68, 123
    mitral, 54, 65–67, 71, 123, 145–146
    pulmonic, 69, 137–138, 140–141, 151
    tricuspid, 69
Stethoscope, 5, 25, 33
Streptococcal infection, 63
Stroke, 116, 129
Sulfadiazine, 64
Supraventricular tachycardia, 79–80
Surgery (*see* Heart surgery)
Sympathetic nervous system:
    alcohol and, 54–55
    amphetamines, 77
    atrial tachycardia, 79–80
    atropine, 23, 79
    blocking agents, 80, 103–104, 118–
    119
    in heart failure, 124–125
Systemic arteries (*see* Arteries)
Systemic circulation, 3, 5–8, 20–23

Systemic veins, 8, 13
Systole, 5, 13, 148
Systolic blood pressure, 5, 91, 109–110, 114, 117–118

Tachycardia:
    atrial, 79–80
    atrial fibrillation, 66, 70–71, 80
    sinus, 78–79
    ventricular, 81–82
    ventricular fibrillation, 81–82, 96, 106
Tetralogy of Fallot, 140–141, 151
Thiazide diuretics, 117–119, 127, 129
Thrill, 28–29
Thrombophlebitis, 10, 71
Thyrotoxicosis, 79, 80
Transposition of the great arteries, 141–142
Transseptal left heart catheterization, 38
Treadmill exercise test, 33
Tricuspid valve, 13–14, 69, 70
Triglyceride levels, 26, 45–47, 56, 89, 98–102, 130

Ultrasound, 26, 34–35

Valve replacement, 147–150
Valves, 13–14
    (*See also* Aortic valve; Mitral valve; Pulmonic valve; Tricuspid valve)

Valvular heart disease, 62, 123, 137–138
Varicose veins, 8
Vein bypass graft, 104–105, 152
Veins:
    pulmonary, 9, 54, 65
    systemic, 8, 13
Vena cavae, 155
Venous blood, 3, 8, 147, 157
Ventricles:
    left, 3, 5, 9, 28, 32, 38–39, 67–69, 96, 123, 134–135
    right, 3, 9, 35–36, 69, 75, 125, 137–138
Ventricular arrhythmias, 76–77, 81–82
Ventricular asystole, 82, 96, 106
Ventricular contraction, 5, 13–14, 148
Ventricular extrasystoles, 76–78
Ventricular fibrillation, 81–82, 96, 106
Ventricular filling, 148
Ventricular premature beats, 76–77
Ventricular septal defect, 39, 139–141, 151
Ventricular septum, 39, 139–141, 154
Ventricular tachycardia, 81–82
Vitamin E, 49

Weight reduction, 47–49
Wolff-Parkinson-White syndrome, 80

X-ray of the chest, 25